Beyond benign neglect:
Early childhood care,
development and nutrition
in metropolitan Lagos, Nigeria

Beyond benign neglect:
Early childhood care, development and nutrition in metropolitan Lagos, Nigeria

Tade Akin Aina
Ibinabo Agiobu-Kemmer
F. Ebam Etta
Marian F. Zeitlin
Kelebogile Setiloane

Produced by the Tufts University School of Nutrition
for the Italian Ministry of Foreign Affairs
and UNICEF, New York

m a l t h o u s e 𝒳𝒫

Malthouse Press Limited

Lagos, Benin, Ibadan, Jos, Oxford, Port-Harcourt, Zaria

Malthouse Press Limited
43 Onitana Street, Off Stadium Hotel Road
Off Western Avenue, Surulere, Lagos
E-mail: malthouse_press@yahoo.com
malthouse_lagos@yahoo.co.uk
Tel: +234 (01) -773 53 44; 0802 364 2402

First published 2008
© Tufts University School of Nutrition 2008
ISBN 978 023 205 2

Distributors:
African Books Collective Ltd
Oxford OX2 0DP, United Kingdom
Email: abc@africanbookscollective.com
Website: http://www.africanbookscollective.com

Preface

This book presents a detailed empirical report of a set of studies and interventions carried out between 1988 and 1991 by a collaborative research team from the Faculty of Social Sciences, University of Lagos and the Tufts University School of Nutrition with the sponsorship of the Joint Nutrition Support Programme of the Italian Government and UNICEF New York. Concerned with the general theme of positive deviance in child development, it focused on early childhood education and development, nutritional practices and values, child rearing values and practices and of course the role and place of the social and cultural context in determining outcomes related to these variables. Te collaborative nature of the work involved partnerships not only between faculty staff but also graduate students who served as Research Assistants and project coordinators. Collaboration in this project was carried out in its true sense with all members of the team made up of sociologists, psychologists, nutritional experts and statistical and quantitative experts all engaged in the design of research methodologies and instruments, the processes of data collection and analyses and the often ponderous and iterative sessions of discussing findings, literature reviews and debating and contesting analyses and conclusions. In this sense, collaboration was ahead of the typical Northern and Southern institutions' project style that is often characterized by an asymmetry of power relations and access to knowledge and its products. Indeed, two of the authors of this book who were research assistants and supervisors have since gained their doctoral degrees with work on materials and related issues gathered from the project. Many more have their Masters. It was indeed an early exercise in mutual counterpart development and capacity building.

Although the publication of the findings have been delayed owing to circumstances beyond the team's control, there is still a lot of currency in the findings of the study, the issues it confronted, the conclusions it drew and even the omissions and silences that it contains. Its engagement with the problem and process of transition (in the case of Nigeria, often partial or/and blocked transition) in social values, norms, institutions and practices around child development, early childhood education, nutrition and family relations still have implications for work in gender relations, family, citizenship, HIV/AIDS, food security and adoption of and adaptation to new technologies and knowledge systems. This recognition of the relevance and currency of the issues informed this publication.

In conclusion, it is important to acknowledge the support and contributions of a wide array of players to the success of this project. These include the former Dean of the Faculty of Social Sciences, University of Lagos, Professor Tomori, all the staff of the Project, the guides and informants in Makoko, Iwaya and the villages in Ogun State, the communities studied and the families that served as research subjects and partners over a period of about two years. It is also important to acknowledge the support of the relevant staff of UNICEF, Lagos particularly Mrs Abosede Akinware and those of the Nigeria Educational Research and Development Council (NERDC). It is as a result of the multiple support, sacrifice and cooperation of all these players that the material presented in this book was put together.

Tade Akin Aina
Project Director, 1988-1991
Nairobi Kenya
August 2005

Table of contents

Section III
The field report

Section I

Introduction

Chapter 1

Introduction

The research and action programme titled *Positive Deviance in Nutrition and Child Development* has been sponsored through the Tufts University School of Nutrition by UNICEF New York and the Joint Nutrition Support Programme of the Italian Government and was carried out in three countries — Nicaragua, Indonesia, and Nigeria — over a period of four years.

In each country, the project had three phases. Phase I was made up of field research. Phase II involved design of action programmes and materials based on the results of Phase I, while Phase III implemented the programmes designed by Phase II.

The Nigerian collaborative project, entitled *Child Development for the Computer Age*, focusing on preschool children, was conducted in Lagos and Ogun States by the Faculty of Social Sciences, University of Lagos in conjunction with Tufts and as part of UNICEF's Child Development Project in Nigeria.

This text presents results of the cross-sectional survey, ethnographic study and psychological testing conducted during Phase I of the Nigerian project.

Central to the project were the concepts of *positive deviance* in nutrition (Zeitlin *et al.*, 1990) and *resilience* in psychology (Werner and Smith, 1982). These terms refer to the phenomenon which occurs in every low-income and deprived community whereby some children grow and develop normally in spite of the observed limitations of their environment, while many other children suffer ill-health, developmental delays, and problems of social adjustment. The methodology assumes that in a given culture and environment, practices of child rearing exist which are based on positive and sometimes brilliant adaptation to the economic and cultural environment.

The purpose of studying success despite adversity was ultimately to apply the factors enabling such success to mobilization programmes, through education and material assistance benefiting children at high risk of malnutrition and cognitive deficits. This is a potentially important approach in developing countries where economic development is occurring too slowly or is often affected by national policies so that it cannot effectively transform the overall living conditions of the poor in the short term. Even during sustainable and equitable socioeconomic development, knowledge of existing effective child-rearing practices should help to utilize resources and empower families.

Qualitative investigations during the study design period centred this research on secular changes in child care with respect to the uses of food and information in the socialization of children, and with respect to changing family structure. In-depth interviews, focus groups and the ethnographic study deepened our understanding of the importance of these aspects of the child's experience.

Practices and beliefs regarding the use of food restriction for the moral training of the child are a particular focus of the research, which finds that the more urban families have relatively more indulgent practices which are associated with better growth and higher cognitive test scores of the children, after adjusting for the minor differences in socioeconomic status in our low-income sample.

This study reports associations between current growth status and current cognitive test performance of 211 children close to the age of two years, the age at which the rate of malnutrition in Nigeria has been found to be highest (Federal Government of Nigeria and UNICEF, 1990).[1]

For the purposes of the study, the link between nutritional status and cognitive test scores permitted us to group the children so as to search for success factors which predict both good growth and good cognitive performance in children emerging from the critical weaning period. These associations confirm that the same children targeted for nutrition intervention should also simultaneously be targeted for cognitive stimulation.

---

[1] It should be noted, however, that our cross-sectional research methods were not designed to quantify the associations between malnutrition and mental development more generally or in the longer term. Conclusions concerning the size of the effects that malnutrition may (or may not) have on the later cognitive functioning of the children cannot be drawn from this research. Prior scientific work in this area indicates that early malnutrition may indeed have subtle long-term implications for mental performance but that not all malnourished children are affected and that it is possible to compensate for nutritional deficits through increased cognitive stimulation.

Organization of the book

This book opens with a fair amount of detail of social background information on the study area and its culture, and proceeds to describe the sample of low income households in Lagos State, Nigeria.

The sections on ecological and social background of the Nigerian study are more comprehensive than similar sections in the other two Phase I reports from Nicaragua and Indonesia, because:

1. Nigerian culture appears to be significantly more different than either the Nicaraguan or Indonesian cultures from the North American and European cultures on which most of our reference literature is based. The Nicaraguan population, for example, is predominantly of European origin.
2. Four of these cultural differences emerge from our study as important to nutritional and developmental outcomes:
   - the very high value placed on fertility,
   - polygamous family structures,
   - the postpartum taboo on sexual relations during breastfeeding, and
   - the use of foods in the moral training of children.

High fertility and polygamy emerge from our study as constituting some constraints to the nutritional status and cognitive performance of urban Nigerian children. Cultural characteristics pertaining to population control and family structure appear to differ in Africa from the pattern that exists in other areas of the world including Asia, Europe, and Latin America (Caldwell and Caldwell 1990). In particular, the cultural taboo on sexual relations during lactation, which traditionally guaranteed birth spacing while reinforcing polygamy, is yielding to premature weaning with shortened birth intervals, increased fertility, and deteriorating nutritional status.

Concern among certain groups that giving the child free access to high quality foods and to food in general — even the breast — will lead to spoiling or moral degradation of the child also has been hinted by our study as a possible cause of malnutrition among the sample age group. The limitation of food as a part of the process of moral training in Nigeria has its parallel in the North American and European practice of leaving infants and young children alone to cry for fear that picking them up or giving them attention will spoil their moral character.

Given that a topic as complex and value-laden as moral training is raised, this study must enter in considerable depth into the culture of child rearing in these parts of Nigeria.

This twelve chapter text is presented in three sections:

Section I comprises chapters 1 and 2 which introduce the study goals and describe the methodology.

Section II provides in three chapters a detailed account of the Yoruba of South-western Nigeria, the population of study. In chapter 3, the culture, society and economy of the Yoruba are discussed. Child care and rearing practices which impinge upon child development are the main focus of chapter 4 while chapter 5 discusses nutrition among the Yoruba.

The field results are reported in section III. The section consists of six chapters, chapter 6 through 11 which discuss the findings in respect of socio-economic, demographic and reproductive characteristics. The household, child care structure, health, sanitation, nutrition and mental development of the sample are also examined.

The concluding section comprising of one chapter, chapter 12, explores the interactional aspects of child care.

Conceptual framework and hypotheses

Underlying assumptions

Under current conditions of poverty and stagnation in the economic development process there is a direct and negative impact of food insecurity, lack of early childhood educational materials, and lack of adequate health and educational facilities all of which negatively affect children's growth and development.

Additionally, it was observed that the development of African children studied is threatened by the gap between the traditional cultural value systems of their grandparents' generation and the survival conditions of the modern era. This puts certain survival requirements of the past in conflict with some of the survival requirements of the present and future.

Adaptiveness of parenting behaviour

The view of LeVine *et al.* (1990) that differences in child development between Africa and the West result from systematic differences in parental strategies of caring for and investing in children was found, to some extent, to be acceptable. These differences in parental practice with regard to child care and stimulation have been linked to a theoretical base (LeVine, 1974; Levine *et al.*, 1988). Their theoretical premise can be summarized in the statement that child-rearing practices are fine-tuned to prepare children to survive and succeed within the rules of the socioeconomic structure which is familiar to their parents.

Accordingly, parents are quick to change their treatment of young children as they perceive new futures for them. LeVine *et al.* (1991) have documented in several populations around the world a spontaneous shift in maternal behaviour away from soothing the infant toward stimulating and teaching him or her, as mothers themselves become educated and set education goals for their children. These shifts are linked to the dramatically changed demands of former agriculturally-based societies, compared to the new information-based society which dominates world markets.

Extending adaptive theories to nutrition

Within this theoretical framework, little attention has yet been given to exploring systematic shifts in nutritional behaviours which occur in response to modernizing trends — shifts which correspond to the changes in child stimulation documented by the LeVines. Research indicating the presence of such shifts was conducted by Guldan (1988). This observational study of 185 four- to 27-month-old Bangladesh infants found that mothers who had been to school were significantly more likely to structure their infant's feeding environment, to supervise feeding actively, and to give more feedings per hour observed than mothers who had no schooling.

Benign neglect

Traditional infant feeding practices sometimes produce negative outcomes for individual children and may lead to the marginal malnutrition of the majority of toddlers, as documented among the Vanatai of Papua New Guinea (Lepowsky 1985). Cassidy (1980; 1987) articulates cultural reasons for child feeding practices which lead to the malnutrition and death of toddlers in traditional societies, but does not enter into the dynamics of secular change. Benign neglect is defined by Cassidy as "parental-caretaker actions supported by customs and beliefs which limit toddler access to the food supply and thereby indirectly potentiate weaning stress and malnutrition, but do so with the benevolent goals of promoting social congruity and normal socialization of the child" (Cassidy 1980).

Cassidy attributes benign neglect to two adaptive responses to chronic scarcity, which she views as inescapable. First, because parents are so stressed by poverty and excess fertility that they must let some of their children die. Their cultures have evolved negative weaning and health practices supported by traditions that permit parents to believe that they are doing their best for their children while actually permitting them to die. Practices which sanction negative outcomes for individual children may be considered historically to be cultural responses to excess population pressure.

Cassidy's second underlying condition for benign neglect is chronic scarcity. She develops the position that the malnourishment of the toddler is a necessary means of socializing and physically adapting children to *limited good*, in societies in which individuals must be physically adapted to survive on low levels of food and in which this food must preferentially be allocated to the most viable and productive family members (Cassidy 1987). Cassidy contrasts the "adaptor's" assumption of limited good with an "activist position" that she claims is based on a false assumption of *unlimited good*. Although of some explanatory power, one must handle Cassidy's motion of `benign neglect' with great care particularly when dealing with societies like those of the Yoruba where children and childbearing are central to the conception of life and social reproduction. 'Benign neglect' in such contexts cannot be the product of conscious decision or action but must be structurally determined to the extent that it is an 'involuntary' act.

Beyond benign neglect

The present study entered in depth into the role of food in the socialization of the child under conditions of limited good in traditional Yoruba society. We also considered the dynamics of change through urbanization and other measures of modernization. In this investigation we positioned ourselves in a participatory activist role which does not assume unlimited good. We assumed rather, that "good" remains highly "limited" but that the manner in which food and attention/information are used by modernizing families to compete for this good has shifted. The activist position of our study seeks to strengthen cultural transitions that are already occurring in response to the changing social and economic reward structure in which limited good is obtainable.

Conceptual framework and hypotheses

In studying positive deviance in both child growth and development, the broad goal of the Nigerian Phase I research was to uncover factors that promote the future success of Nigerian children in an era of advanced technology. Objectives under this goal included the discovery of specific child care factors, as specified in the hypotheses below. They also included the search for the emerging perceptions of childhood and family life that support the investment of needed resources in the children.

Conceptual framework

The conceptual framework of the study (fig. 1.1) posits that socioeconomic characteristics (left column), household and community demographic characteristics (right) influence child care variables and child outcomes (centre). Each column is divided into a primary component (above) and a cultural distance component (below). Arrows in this framework signify main hypotheses.

Primary hypotheses

The study's primary research hypotheses for child development concern characteristics identified through review of the literature (Zeitlin, Ghassemi and Mansour, 1990). Our interest in testing these hypotheses is to discover the kinds of care and other resources that are most highly associated with good outcomes. The primary hypotheses are as follows:

(1) The household's economic and educational resources (left column) and the family and community structure in which child care is provided (right column) will determine child development as measured simultaneously by good growth status and good cognitive performance (centre column). Exposure to modernizing influences (cultural distance) will be closely linked to socioeconomic status.
Important structural characteristics of the household will include the mother's support from her husband and other family members and her reproductive burden.
2) These influences will operate through child care, which includes the quality of child feeding, health behaviours, and home stimulation and psychological attunement.

Fig 1.1: Conceptual framework for Nigerian survey analysis

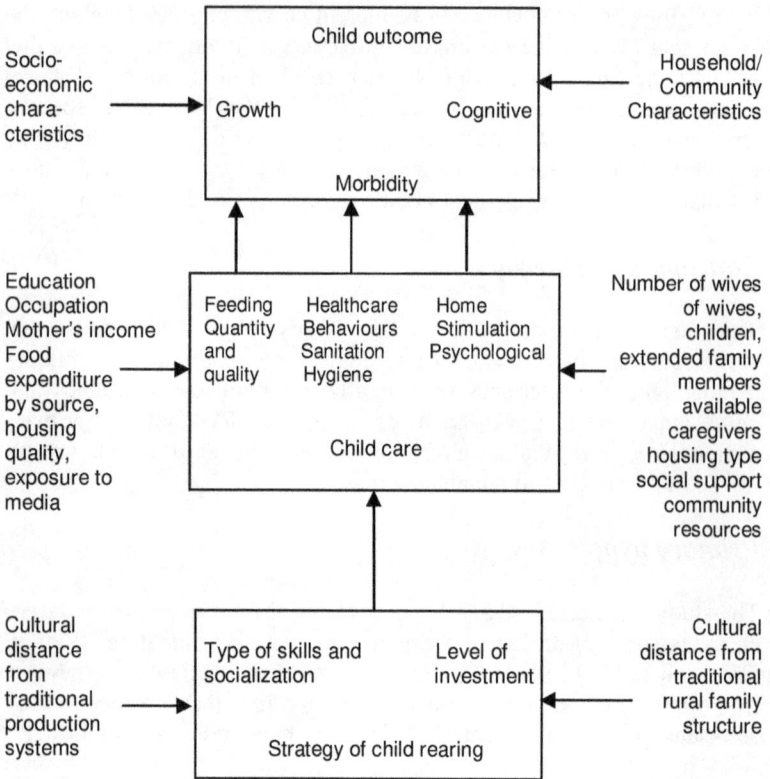

3) These intervening variables will be significantly associated with good development of the child.

Specific hypotheses investigated were:

1) The mother's working conditions will be related to the nutritional status and cognitive test scores of the children. The less time she must leave the child the better.
2) Child care by family members over six years of age, grandmothers, and maids will be associated with better outcomes than care by the

mother's female friends and children under six, or by multiple secondary caretakers.

3) Higher scores on the psychological variables measuring the warmth, stimulation, and encouragement given by the mother to the child will be associated with better child outcomes.

Cultural research hypotheses

It is because the cultural research hypotheses of a study of this nature are far from obvious that the study team undertook the in-depth qualitative investigations of cultural factors reported in sections three to five. The cultural hypotheses are:

1) Cultural distance both from traditional production systems (bottom left column, fig. 6.1) and from traditional family and community structures (bottom right column) will be associated with increased likelihood of good child development, as measured simultaneously by growth status and cognitive test scores.

In other words, families who have made two transitions will have better child outcomes. The first transition is away from reliance on traditional seniority networks and traditional occupations for present and future economic security. The second is away from the concept of unlimited good in child bearing and a family structure of self-supporting wives in a polygamous unit.

We should emphasize, however, that distance from traditional African culture does not imply recommendation of the adoption of aspects of traditional Eurasian culture that may also be ill suited to modern economic productivity. The cloistered, relatively non-productive role of Eurasian women, for example, may once have been necessary to assure the legitimacy and survival of heirs to landholdings. However, it is ill adapted to modern economic systems and not an adequate model for Africa. Definitely there are aspects of traditional culture that favour greater psychological and other forms of integration in the modern world in which we live.

Positive effects should be apparent so long as the cultural distance follows a positive path, i.e. after controlling for primary socioeconomic and child care variables. Distance *away from* may imply distance *toward* something else. This "something else" may take a variety of forms. The goal of the study was to investigate these forms inductively rather than deductively through model testing.

2) Cultural distance effects will operate through the type of socialization given to the child, the types of skills valued and taught, and the level of investment of resources in the child. The child care variables which measure type of socialization and level of investment are included among the measurements of feeding, health behaviours and home stimulation.
3) As in the case of the primary hypotheses, these cultural influences will operate through the child care variables; and
4) These child care variables will be significantly associated with good development of the child.

The specific hypotheses in respect of cultural influence were:

1) Children with higher nutritional status will have significantly higher cognitive test scores.
2) Two-year-old children who score relatively higher in performing household chores will score lower in mental development index, reflecting the different socialization priorities of their parents.
3) Women with no primary caretakers for the child other than themselves will have poor child outcomes. Since only one percent of this sample are non-earning housewives, the productive work levels of all women make an alternative source of child care other than the mother indispensable to good outcomes.
4) Short birth intervals, reflecting abandonment of the post-partum taboo on sexual relations without effective contraception, will prevent improvements in growth and cognitive performance that should otherwise be associated with increased education of the parents. As higher parental education will lead to shorter birth intervals, these will negatively affect growth and development, cancelling out the beneficial effects of greater parental education.
5) The child's Mental Development Index (MDI), reflecting his or her psychological rapport with the parent and hence access to food, will appear in the analysis as a stronger determinant of growth status than growth status as a determinant of MDI.
6) Among the foods investigated, greatest reporter bias will attach to distribution of meat, because of its symbolic role in socializing children. In addition, maternal child health (MCH) nurses may give conflicting advice regarding meat, either recommending meat for malnourished children or reinforcing the traditional belief that meat causes worms. This bias will result in inconsistencies in the data.

7) There will be consistent associations between the strength of the stated belief that meat causes the moral degradation of the child, the degree of restriction on high prestige foods (particularly of animal origin) given to the child, and the growth status and mental development scores of the child.

8) The reliance on restriction of meat and of food in general for moral training will decrease significantly with maternal education, wealth, and urbanization.

9) Greatest ambivalence and reporter bias attaches to distribution of meat in particular, and will result in inconsistencies in the data.

10) Given deep-rooted resistance to changing the distribution of both food and information, although information and stimulation practices start to change more readily than food distribution practices, they must traverse greater cultural distance in order to empower children to become technologically competitive. Redistribution of food encounters more initial resistance, but its achievement requires fewer new skills of parents.

11) Appeal to parents' desire for their children's school achievement is an effective entry point for change, as it presents the children's needs in a context dissociated from the traditional distribution system.

12) Mothers closest to and most dependent on the traditional production system and traditional social networks are most careful to ration food, censor information, and mould their children to group norms.

13) Verbal interactions and information exchange between parents and children increase in quantity and change in quality as families rely less on traditional seniority structures for their present and future livelihoods.

14) Religious membership and the nature of religious beliefs regarding entitlement of individuals to information, power, and divine protection may influence information transfer to young children.

15) Because religion and healing were not separate in traditional society, the mental associations that people still have between the two domains may make it particularly effective to enlist the church and the mosque in child rearing, nutrition, and health education.

Tested hypotheses

1) The physical development index (PDI) scores will be higher than mental development index (MDI) scores of the study children.

2) Two-year-old children who score relatively higher in performing household chores will score lower in mental development index, after controlling for other factors.
3) The child's Bayley Mental Development Index (MDI), reflecting his or her psychological characteristics and hence access to food, will appear in the analysis as a stronger determinant of growth status than will growth status or Physical Development Index (PDI).

Ethnography

The research included an ethnographic study of ten thousand households with six of the highest and four of the lowest-scoring children on the Bayley Scales of Infant Development (Aina *et al.*).

Prior to the survey and throughout the intervention, the project team carried out in-depth interviews with opinion leaders and periodic focus groups with community parents and grandparents and with faculty, staff and students at the University of Lagos.

Chapter 2

Methodology

Site and sample selection

This study focused primarily on urban and semi-rural children in Lagos State, Southwestern Nigeria, with a small rural sub-sample. Because of the difficulties of comparison across different ethnic groups, only Yoruba children were selected. Two-year-olds were chosen because these children still reflect the nutritional experience of the weaning process, yet at the same time have started to display verbal and certain other cognitive skills predicting school performance. The high malnutrition rate among two-year-olds in Nigeria (Federal Government of Nigeria and UNICEF, 1990) also makes this a good age at which to detect determining factors. At this age active growth monitoring is expected.

The rural and semi-rural settlements selected included six small rural villages and two medium-sized semi-rural towns in Ifo-Otta Local Government Authority (LGA). The rural villages were situated on an almost unsettled area at some distance from the main Lagos - Abeokuta road, about 45 minutes from Lagos by vehicle. The semi-rural settlements bordered this road, about an hour to an hour and a half from Lagos.

The urban settlement was the predominantly low-income settlement of Makoko in Metropolitan Lagos.

Eligibility for selection as a study family in the cross-sectional field study included the following specifications:

        (a) mother is Yoruba,

        (b) child is 22 to 26 months old,

        (c) child is not a twin,

(d) child has a birth certificate to verify age, and

(e) both mother and child are present.

The last two requirements automatically eliminated from our sample high-risk children who were fostered with grandmothers or others living in households lacking records such as birth certificates.

Sample size for the cross-sectional field research totalled 211, including a census sample of 181 mothers and their children and an additional purposive sample of 30 households screened for the presence of a malnourished child in order to better understand the problems associated with malnutrition.

Instruments

The survey instruments which were administered by a team of two field workers during home visits of approximately three hours' duration, include the following:

1) A 52-item food frequency questionnaire for current consumption, diet histories for infancy and weaning, questions about the family meal schedule, and maternal attitudes related to food beliefs and practices.
   The research team of the University of Lagos first wrote the questionnaires in English and pre-tested them using informal Yoruba translations. They then translated them into Yoruba for further pre-testing before the wording, codes, and procedures were finalized.
2) Structured observations of feeding, play, and teaching sessions of the mother and child.
3) The Bayley Scales of Infant Development (Bayley, 1969), supplemented with interviewer-rated scales of behaviour and affect of the mother and child.
4) A socio-demographic questionnaire and a modified Caldwell H.O.M.E. inventory (Caldwell and Bradley, 1984).
5) Anthropometric measurements including weights, heights, and mid-upper arm circumference of the children, and weights and heights of the mothers.

Data collection and management

Birth dates were from birth certificates, weights were taken to the nearest

0.1 kg using a hanging scale with a capacity of 25 kg. A wooden stadiometre built by the project was used to measure height in centimetres (2-6 years).

Raw weights and heights were converted to Z-scores of the NCHS-WHO standards (Lavoipierre, 1983) using software provided by the United States Centre for Disease Control (CDC). Two centimetres were added to the standing heights of the children just below two years, whose measurements were treated by the CDC programme as recumbent lengths.

The data were recorded on pre-coded forms which were checked for error within 24 hours of collection. Interviewers were sent back to the field to complete missing records.

A Tufts University master's-level nutritionist co-supervised the data collection. She contributed to training the interviewers and standardized their anthropometric measurement methods as recommended by WHO (Lavoipierre, 1983).

Data analysis

The data were analysed at Tufts University with the Statistical Package for the Social Sciences (SPSSX 1988) and SAS (1985) and in Nigeria using SPSS-PC on the project's microcomputer.

The richness of the data and the goal of identifying hitherto unknown relationships led us to use the full range of multivariate approaches to explore the data including factor analysis, ordinary least-squares regression, two-stage least-squares regression, and logistic regression contrasting children who were high on both nutrition and mental development scores with children who were low on both upon which a substantial part of the report is based.

The approach to data analysis combined exploration and theory construction with hypothesis testing. A vast number of psychosocial and physiological factors have been linked to the nutritional status of young children and can equally be associated with their cognitive test performance (Zeitlin, Ghassemi and Mansour 1990, pp 36-72). This body of theory hypothesizes potentially significant associations between growth status and cognitive performance of the Nigerian children and every variable in the data set.

Assumptions in the design of the study were that:

1) many but not all of the hypothesized factors would be significant;

2) among significant factors some but not all could be measured sensitively enough to permit detection of the significant associations;
3) particularities in cultural behaviour and the physical environment would determine the forms in which expected associations would be manifested; and
4) thorough data exploration would be needed to attempt to model the inherent relationships.

Dependent variables

Nutritional status and developmental test outcomes were kept distinct in relation to variables hypothesized to influence them directly, and for comparison with each other. However, we combined these outcomes for major analyses because our goal was to discover the factors that promote overall development of the child. The well-developing child shows good growth and good cognitive performance simultaneously.

Logistic regressions contrast children in the top third for both growth and cognitive development with those in the bottom third (N=69 in both groups: Table 7.1). With a few exceptions, the high-high group are children whose cognitive test score was above the median of 91, whose height-for-age Z-score (HAZ) was above -2.25, and whose weight-for-height Z-score (WHZ) was above -1.25. The low-low group had all three scores below these levels.

Exceptions were made for children who were borderline for height but very high for MDI and vice versa. Most such children with high MDI scores were classified with the high-high group, on the logic that the nutrients they were receiving were adequate to permit superior performance. Table 7.1 shows the growth and developmental mean values of all outcome indicators for the high and low groups.

To create a continuous combined variable for analysis, the SPSSX (1988) Z-score program was applied to weight-for-age, height-for-age, and MDI scores. The new anthropometric Z-scores were averaged, and this average was in turn averaged with the new MDI Z-score. For this continuous variable the two anthropometric scores were used in order to factor in a hypothesized ceiling on overall growth caused by overall food restriction (WAZ) and an additional ceiling on linear growth caused by specific restriction of animal foods (HAZ). This positive deviance variable was given the name ZPOSDEV1.

Other composite variables

The construction of the variables will be presented in the sections in which they are reported. While most composite variables are entirely theory-based, some were constructed in a manner that reflected associations in the data, where such associations were consistent with the theoretical constructs guiding the research.

In a large and rich data set this process of fitting variables and refining and pre-testing hypotheses can continue almost indefinitely. In most cases, however, major associations become visible early in the analysis.

We give attention here to operationalizing the uniquely cultural concepts, which may be less familiar to the reader. These concepts are:

1) Cultural distance from reliance on traditional seniority networks and traditional occupations for the family's present and future economic security.

Variables:
- family's exposure and commitment to modern schooling:
  - mother's and father's schooling
  - schooling of mother's parents
- mother's exposure to television and radio and knowledge of current events
- family's distance from traditional agriculture:
  - whether mother, father, mother's father or grandfather farmed

2) Cultural distance from the concept of unlimited good in child bearing and a family structure of self-supporting wives in a polygamous unit.

Variables:
- family structure and economic organization:
  - number of wives
  - number of father's children by other wives
  - presence of father
  - father mentioned as child's caretaker
  - ratio of mother's income to father's contribution toward food expenditure

– limitation of family size:
  - number of additional children wanted by mother
  - mother practices family planning, currently or ever
  - duration of breast-feeding
  - average birth interval
– housing type:
  - face-to-face dwelling
  - persons per room
– membership in religion with monogamous values:
  - Muslim versus Christian (too few in the sample still adhere to traditional religion for stratified analysis)

3) Increase in quantity and change in quality of verbal interactions and information exchange between parents and children.

Variables:
  – investment in home stimulation of the child
    - books, manufactured toys, place for child's own possessions
    - verbal interaction, playing with child
    - free expression of praise or encouragement to child

4) Changes in type of training interaction.

Variables:
  - more teaching of "ABC-123" (a local term for basic alphabet and counting skills)
  - fewer chores performed by two-year-old

5) Shift from food restriction for child's training to investment for child's development.

Variables:
  - attitudes toward meat and moral training, stealing, and scarcity,
  - frequency of eating animal foods, fruits, and snacks
  - portion sizes of meat that mother would allocate as a measure of her personal interpretation of the seniority distribution function
  - duration of bottle feeding

6) Investment in health behaviours.

Variables:
- child is taken outside home for treatment of fever
- source of treatment is modern health worker
- modern hygiene and sanitation

Categories used in reporting

The descriptive statistics display the values of all variables by rural, semi-rural, and urban location. This set of comparisons uses the systematic sample of 180 children (excluding one child with an ambiguous location code). It excludes the purposive sub-sample of malnourished children of whom 10 were urban and 20 semi-rural.

Statistically significant contrasts are also reported between the families of children falling in the high-high versus the low-low developmental categories. Both the systematic and purposive samples are represented in developmental status contrasts. Both samples are also included in multivariate analyses except when location enters the analyses.

Ethnographic methods

The research included an ethnographic study of ten households with six of the highest and four of the lowest-scoring children on the Bayley's Scales of Infant Development (Aina *et al.*). The ethnographic sub-component of the study involved several hours of close observations (both unobtrusive and participant), interviews and interventions.

A field ethnographer visited ten families, five from urban and five from semi-rural homes, over a seven month period. Through observation of the household and informal interviews with the mothers, she gathered data on the nutritional aspects of home life such as how much and what kinds of foods were eaten regularly and aspects of the home environment likely to affect child cognitive development such as the verbal interaction between the mother and child during the day and the amount of sensory and motor stimulation to which the child was exposed. It was also intended, through informal interviews, to consider the mother's perception of the possibilities open to her in her life and her ideas about her child's ability to succeed.

Intervention

As well as providing a means of collecting in-depth data about the mothers' child rearing practices, the ethnography was intended to be an interventionary tool for the project. Through conversations with the mother, the ethnography intended to discover aspects of mothers' lifestyles and ways of thinking which could be obstacles in the way of eventually getting them to feed their children adequately and prepare them for school. These conversations, which we called interventionary conversations, were supposed to commence after the ethnographer had established a thorough acquaintance with the family, and to continue during the remainder of her data gathering period. She also was to suggest alternate ways of child rearing to the mother, stressing the importance of sufficient protein in the diet and of intellectual stimulation.

Collecting data on the mothers' responses to new ideas was one way in which the project hoped to get an idea of the cognitive, psychological and pragmatic obstacles that stand in the way of improved child rearing. In addition to the conversations, the interventionary aspect of the ethnography also was to include trials of new procedures and referrals for various conditions.

In practice, however, whatever intervention that occurred was indirect being the product of mothers being exposed to new knowledge and approaches as a result of interaction and rapport between them and the ethnographer. The ethnographer did not try direct interventions which might jeopardize her ongoing relationships with the mothers during the study.

Ethnographic sample procedure

From the results of the larger survey, the highest urban MDI was 130 while the lowest was 7.6. The highest semi-rural MDI was 124, while the lowest was 50.

Using this range of scores, six of the highest and four of the lowest subjects were selected for the detailed ethnographic sub-study. Several malnourished children were excluded from the sample as being too untypical. So also were the first group of children visited at the beginning of the survey, so as to eliminate the factor of the testers' initial unfamiliarity with test instruments. The children scoring 50 and 130 belonged to these groups and hence were excluded.

The mother of the index child, whether a high or a low scorer, should if possible also have another younger baby, and preferably an older sibling between the ages of four and ten. It was felt that this would permit an ethnographic inspection of infant feeding at the age when the babies may start to become malnourished. Presence of an older sibling would permit observation of the parent's intellectual stimulation of the child who starts to ask questions and attend school.

The Bayley MDI scores were classified into three broad groups, namely low, average and high scores, for the rural and the urban locations. From within these two sets of samples, the six children who scored high and four children who scored low were selected as follows, with the names changed to protect the privacy of the families. All but one had siblings.

	Urban	*MDI*	*Semi-Rural*	*MDI*
High	Lekan Olusola	121	Olu Apata	122
	Alira Oluwole	115	Kike Jacob	124
	Abbey Sowola	115	Funso Odelami	109
Low	Ayo Qudus	79	Latif Semiu	77
	Kunle Adebo	77	Gani Oludoja	76

A factor worth mentioning in relation to the children's performance on the Bayley is that testers were complete strangers to the children. Allowance must be given for the possibility that the best response might not have been elicited from the children, due to the fact that they were seeing the testers for the first time, although the presence of the mothers during testing was hoped to mitigate this factor.

A total of 240 hours were spent on collecting the ethnographic information reported.

Section II

The Yoruba of south western Nigeria: child care, rearing practices and nutrition

Chapter 3

The Yoruba of south-western Nigeria: culture, society and economy

Introduction

In this section of the book, we explore the cultural and economic underpinnings of practices that limit the food and information provided to young children, and hence may prevent children from reaching their full potential. Why did some traditional Nigerian parents have to rely on rationing their children's food, and withholding animal food, as a means of moral training? Why did they need to ration stimulation and information for the child's own good, so that children were traditionally seen but not heard? We also investigate the factors causing these practices to change in modern Nigeria.

As noted in the introduction, our main reason for applying the positive deviance-psychological resilience research approach to these issues is to understand and if possible facilitate this process of secular transition.

Cultural overview

The Yoruba ethnic group, who are the subjects of this study, make up roughly 20% of the Nigerian population. Yorubaland has the greatest concentration of cities and towns in sub-Saharan Africa, with at least nine cities of more than 100,000 population and a 60%-70% rate of urbanization (Federal Office of Statistics 1986). Lagos, which is the home of our urban sample children, had a population 5.6 million in 1991 according to the provisional figures of the census. Southwestern (Yoruba) Nigeria has the highest concentration of industries in Nigeria, with more than 50% of the country's manufacturing output, predominantly in light industries manufacturing products such as furniture, textiles, wearing apparel, plastics, paper, leather goods, foodstuffs, confectionery, beverages, and tobacco products.

One reason for selecting the Yoruba for a positive deviance and resilience study under conditions of rapid modernization was the advanced level of Yoruba traditional culture. The Yoruba had a complex pre-colonial system of economic production and trade onto which modernization was grafted. Therefore, we assumed it likely that their solutions to problems of modernization might reflect a greater depth of uniquely African tradition than the solutions of peoples who had led technologically simpler lifestyles.

With cities that date from the middle ages, the Yoruba were in part an exception to the Caldwells' generalization regarding rural demographic structure and communal land-ownership in Africa (Caldwell and Caldwell 1990). The Yoruba pre-colonial town crafts were among the earliest developed in Africa (Callaway 1967). Private ownership of land, governed by male primogeniture, had emerged in the Bini Kingdom, but had not replaced clan ownership as the predominant form.

Land belonged to the lineage and was freely available to all lineage members. According to Caldwell and Caldwell (1990) this African pattern is central to the continent's continuing high population growth rate at a time when Asian and Latin American fertility rates are decreasing. The transition from clan ownership to individual ownership of land is claimed to have occurred in most of Europe and Asia about 5,000 years ago. It did not occur in sub-Saharan Africa, however, because ecological conditions did not favour the accumulation of agricultural surplus. Societies in which families traditionally owned their own land are purported to be more easily motivated to limit births to the number that their landholdings or other resources can support. Private ownership did not become the predominant form of land tenure among the Yoruba until the 1960s.

Though land was plentiful, it was laborious to cultivate using swidden, or slash and burn, agricultural methods. Each additional wife and each additional child increased the amount of land that could be cultivated and hence the food security of the domestic unit.

Women were usually subordinate to men, in an asymmetrical relationship in which a man was entitled to exclusive sexual access to his wife and some degree of control over her labour. She did not have reciprocal rights. Each gender had its own age hierarchy, through which individuals could expect to pass as they became older and met local standards of maturity (LeVine *et al.*, 1990).

The cultural norms governing key aspects of society for example,

> economic distribution and management rules governing production, consumption and social services, household and community composition and structure, i.e. the configuration of human and physical resources which were customized to meet the requirements of the production system:

had great force, as social order in traditional African societies was maintained and regulated through shared beliefs and values. Coercion was practiced, but it was predominantly moral persuasion rather than legal pressure (Turnbull, 1974). Indoctrination into the community belief structure started at birth, with the very first ritual act, and continued through childhood with other acts and practices, so that by the time the child had reached puberty, having gone through all the necessary indoctrination, he was a full member of the society.

Economic distribution and management rules

The domestic group operated as a hierarchy of labour in which the least desirable work was delegated downward to women and children, and as a hierarchy of consumption, in which privileges were distributed upwards towards male elders. The youngest children, after weaning, did the most menial tasks, while having the least claim on valued goods, such as meat to eat (LeVine, 1973, pp. 131-133). The daytime care of infants and very young children when the mother was otherwise occupied was delegated primarily to older siblings.

Power, entitlement, and seniority

The main overarching rule was that power and entitlement to resources increased with seniority, and that all formally designated power belonged to the senior partner in any transaction. Junior members increased their levels of security and privilege through informal exchanges of goods and services, and through loyalty and deference to seniors.

Seniors had the responsibility to exercise authority over those junior to them and intercede in their interest. They had, concomitantly, an unquestioned right to command the services of their juniors. These authoritarian management rules, similar to those of the modern military, worked in a continuum from about the age of two years through adulthood. Although seniority systems in other parts of Africa, and perhaps universally, tend to operate on the same principles, the specific conventions differ among cultures. The particular system we studied has the following implications:

Implications for skills training and information transfer

1) High priority was placed on social intelligence
Traditional Yoruba culture gives priority to social intelligence training, which is manipulative and instrumentalist. Studies of traditional peoples in other regions of Africa also have found highest value attached to social intelligence. The value placed upon social skills is expressed in the Yoruba adage: *Ọmọ t'oba m'owo we, a ba agba jeun.* "The child who knows how to wash his hands, will eat with elders." This saying is interpreted to mean that children or younger people who have mastered correct social skills will be entitled to gain privileges otherwise reserved for elders. It also has indirect implications for nutrition.

While attentive to age, seniority among the Yoruba also derived from gender, hereditary titles, designated leadership roles, physical ability, supernatural endowment (as in the case of the priesthood), and marriage conventions which dictated that the new wife was junior to any of her husband's family members born before the date of her marriage (Fadipe 1970). Given the many demands of productive labour, distinctions defining seniority were, of necessity, elaborate in Yoruba culture, expressed in the myriad terms by which individuals greeted and addressed each other. Distinctions among these titles and greetings could claim the same importance now attached in the modern sector to job grades and descriptions, working hours, and salary levels in a monetized service structure. Greetings and small gifts provided the verbal "cash and small change" that were needed to settle interpersonal accounts in the exchange of productive labour and social services.

Upward mobility was accessible through social manipulation and differences in social operating style between subgroups occasional analysis and commentary. According to local cultural stereotypes, the

Oyo Yoruba were the most socially manipulative, whereas Ondo and Ekiti Yoruba were relatively more direct, less hierarchical. The Oyo called their parents by the formal rather than the familiar word for 'you'. According to the stereotype, they expressed anger through passive aggression rather than directly and attacked verbally with sarcasm, irony, and oblique symbolism. By contrast an Ondo Yoruba man would carry his cutlass and threaten to cut off your head.

Under the old socioeconomic structure, it was of primary importance for children to learn correct social greetings and titles and to learn the exchanges of goods and services which were implicit in the child's rank in the hierarchy, or which could be obtained through special merit, etc. Because of their intricacy, the subcomponents of these social skills had to be acquired separately, and much practice was needed to master the necessary variety of their combinations. The University of Lagos team hypothesizes that the complexity of learning to master the social subcomponents and the rules governing their combination in traditional societies matches the complexity of learning the component parts of technical skills required today by the modern economic order. The ethnographic study revealed that certain of the high-scoring children were already adept by the age of two-and-a-half at giving complex social greetings and judging when to use formal versus informal possessive pronouns.

We believe that this cultural difference in the skills required for economic success underlies the differences in parental training of children, starting in infancy.

2) Juniors were forbidden to question seniors

The right to ask questions was always grounded in a "need to know" basis for production-related skills in agriculture, the crafts guilds, and the medical and priestly guilds. Technical information requirements of the workers at the bottom of the traditional seniority system were minimal, since the tasks they performed were relatively repetitive and had fixed sets of rules, requiring few incoming technical instructions. Managers at the top also required little information or feedback from the bottom. The uses of information and misinformation in this management structure differed dramatically from one under a modern monetized and highly technical production system.

Outside of the priestly and medical occupations, the right to question on the basis of the "need to know" was narrowly defined and did not generally extend to current events, general information regarding causality in the physical universe and in the social realm, and other aspects of daily life. The right to ask questions and to be conversant in these areas was a privilege proportionate to increasing seniority. Juniors could not question their seniors because questioning was perceived as defying the rules of the seniority system. In questioning, the junior member of the interaction steps out of the submissive role by requiring something of the senior member, for a question demands an answer. By obliging the senior person to respond, the junior questioner is temporarily attempting to assume command.

Under this system, it was necessary for parents to refuse to answer their children's questions in order to instil in them a proper respect for seniority. Children and other subordinates were to be seen but not heard. Furthermore, the unobtrusively listening child was not permitted to look at the adult speaker's mouth or eyes, and was thereby deprived of visual information.

3) Strategic misinformation was essential to management

Achieving desired social ends depended on certain elements of secrecy and deliberate misinformation. The system could not function if information were freely accessible to those who did not know its rules. Misinformation was essential to the distribution of tasks and to the flow of goods and service.

It was not acceptable for a junior to refuse to do something for a senior person simply because of personal needs or desires to do something else, or because the individual called upon received insufficient personal benefits from the task. It was implicitly understood that the necessary way to reserve time and energy for one's own affairs was to pretend to be absent or unwell when senior persons asked for services, while in fact going about one's personal business.

Untruths thus were necessary social circuit breakers, signalling the need for the senior person either to set someone else on the task or to increase its profitability to the person summoned. Telling lies was always condemned by the senior members of the system. However, some falsification or confusion regarding one's physical movements was accepted as a necessary form of self protection.

The need to protect one's self was intensified by perceived proximity to the world of spirits, and led to withholding of information in the belief that enemies would use it for their own perhaps evil purposes. The old pantheon of Yoruba gods, or *orisha*, is metaphorically similar to the court structure of the ancient Yoruba kingdoms, with a remote high ruler not usually approached directly and a variety of intermediary courtiers, who can be entreated for favours, and expected to engage in intrigue of a sort not necessarily benign.

By contrast, monotheistic Christianity and Islam claim to provide their members with direct access to a single, all-powerful and unquestionably loving spiritual ruler. In these systems the individual may be less susceptible to evil intrigue, and therefore may be able to become more straightforward in giving information about himself and his movements. The "born again" Christian movement, for example, combines a personal experience of salvation and of the presence of Christ with a group commitment to honest and open business practices and telling the truth.

4) *Children had to be strategically misinformed and taught to misinform*

Under the old system, it was necessary for parents to tell untruths to their children in ways that taught the child the futility of asking frivolous questions and prepared him or her for verbal manipulation and survival. Children were also trained to give misleading information by the common task assigned to children of misinforming outsiders about their parents' whereabouts.

Misinformation used by parents to control a child's behaviour included fanciful threats and promises, e.g. the bogeyman (*egungun*) and false promises of rewards of treats, gifts, outings, trips, or visits. Parents could take a playful, gleeful approach to tricking the adversarial child, sometimes with elaborate hoaxes. The child would learn by example. Misinformation included fanciful answers to the child's questions about the physical universe and about social topics not appropriate to his or her age and rank. These answers might be laced with irony and symbolism that the child was expected to gradually master. A caretaker who interacted with the child in this manner was often highly attuned to the child. Such a caretaker was engaging the child in a sophisticated verbal exchange which did not have the purpose of accurate information transfer. The stork, the tooth fairy, and Santa Claus suggest remnants of a similar process of giving children symbolic misinformation in some North American and European cultures.

5) *Perceived personal characteristics weighed heavily in determining a child's well-being*

As indicated in the proverb in (1) above, children as well as adults earned privileges in the hierarchy through good behaviour. Since the stated purpose of food restriction is moral training, if a parent perceives that a child is already trained, she may not need to withhold food strictly and may feel safer in confiding information. One mother in the ethnographic study, proud that her son was not greedy, justified her responsiveness to him by saying that he usually went a long time without asking to eat, so whenever he did ask, she fed him, knowing that if he asked, he must have become very hungry.

The statement that a child's characteristics determine the child's well-being should be tempered with understanding of the different levels at which causality occurs. The mother may react to the child's characteristics, but it is the transactional system between them, in which she is the more powerful member, which determines the outcomes for the child. Some of what the mother perceives to be inherent in the child actually is caused by her treatment of the child.

To cite an extreme example of such perceptions from northeast Brazil, Scheper-Hughes (1987) describes a folk diagnosis made by mothers of "sickness of the child", an incurable wasting condition which signals to the mother that she should withdraw her emotional investment, neglect the child and allow it to die. The mother takes her cues from characteristics of the child — chronic illness, extreme thinness, and listlessness which the mother interprets as a lack of will to live. Yet it is the mother's behaviour in response to the cues that leads to the child's death. In most cases, moreover, the child would not have declined to the point where the mother made this terminal diagnosis if the mother's previous treatment had been satisfactory.

In other cases, e.g. visible birth defects, the child's characteristics may be truly causal (Mull, 1987). Fragmentary but suggestive research along these lines in Nigeria has reported parents of *spina bifida* children defaulting frequently from the hospital and showing relief on the child's demise (Oyewole, 1985). A degree of indifference to their handicapped children was identified among Nigerian fathers (Enwemeka, 1983). Even among health care providers, children with kwashiorkor may provoke depression leading to diminution or evasion of contact with the child (Izuora, 1983).

In traditional Yoruba culture, divination on the third day after birth commonly set the elders' perceptions of and expectations of a child. While this practice has declined, divinatory revelations regarding the child's nature and destiny are not uncommon. Children may be perceived to be reincarnations of grandparents, for example, in a reincarnational model that is similar to the model in Northern European Jewish folk culture, in which more than one child can reincarnate the same ancestor because the uniqueness of the soul is not reincarnated. This reincarnation belief differs from that of the Ibos of Eastern Nigeria, in which the unique individual can be reborn seven times, and may wilfully return to be with loved ones or seek revenge for wrongs during the earlier life. Reporting on informal observations, the field workers of the present study noted that perceived resemblances to ancestors or relatives influenced mothers' reactions to children.

Challenges and resources for transition

1) Misinformation has negative effects in modern settings

In the current transition from traditional patterns, parents wish their children to excel in school and in technical capability. Yet giving the child misinformation regarding technical matters slow down the learning of correct information. It also tends to delay mastery of logical thinking, since at an early age the child is expected to accept, as true, explanations that are logically inconsistent with what he or she perceives and knows from other sources.

In a fully monetized system, and even more critically in a complex computerized system, the circuit-breaking function of misinformation — a function valuable in the former production system — sabotages the operation of the new information- and communications-based system. Moreover, as services become monetized, it is no longer necessary or possible to oblige people to perform at no charge duties which they used to be able to escape only by strategic misinformation. Thus, the former uses of misinformation become increasingly irrelevant and dysfunctional in the newer system.

2) Accelerated inflow of new information is needed

Because the production and service systems are so much more complex in modern society, the total amount of information to be mastered is greater than in traditional society. Rapid mastery of new information must continue over the course of a lifetime. Therefore children need to start learning early, and the speed with which new information is given them needs to be increased. In industrialized societies it has been estimated that children learn an average of five new words per day through much of early childhood. Children have such capacity to learn that their speed of learning is limited mainly by the rate at which the information is presented to them.

3) A traditional model exists for senior-junior parity in entitlement to information

A model for a teaching relationship between adults and children which gave children a form of peer status with their elders existed in traditional society. The Ifa priesthood of traditional healers requires the memorization and mastery of voluminous oral texts and traditions. Interviews with two Ifa priests who trained child apprentices disclosed that the traditional priests were well aware that strict maintenance of the age hierarchy system was incompatible with such training (Chief Atanda, personal communication, 1989).

Only children destined by divination or whose early characteristics conformed to those expected of potential priests would be apprenticed. From the start of training, as early as the age of two (but often later), the child destined to become a priest was given the honorary status of an elder, so that all information and explanations could be made available to him or her. A rule of training was that the apprentice's questions were answered truthfully in full.

One chief illustrated this point with the story of his own eight-year-old son who had been apprenticed to the Ifa from early childhood. The boy approached the headmaster of his elementary school and informed him that he was a *babalawo*, or Ifa priest, and that therefore the teachers had to treat him with respect. The headmaster's response was to send round to the house to find out if this were true, and then to inform the teachers that they must accord the boy the seniority he requested.

This seniority status was, however, not extended to food distribution. As stated by one informant, "We don't spoil them with food." The frequent animal sacrifices to the *Ifa*, however, assured a meat supply to priestly households. Some ceremonies for child apprentices also required them to eat the flesh of the animals whose powers they were to incorporate by ritual means.

Five of the six families of high-scoring children and none among the four low scorers in the ethnographic study demonstrated sharing of information from parents to children that more resembled a peer relationship than a hierarchical relationship. The mother who was most noted for sharing her thoughts, answering children's questions, and explaining her activities happened to be a devout member of the Jehovah's Witnesses, a group whose emphasis on the individual's responsibility to "witness" may create a point of view corresponding to a priestly role in society. This mother was observed to give her two-year-old a careful explanation of where she was taking the baby sister, why, and who would be caring for the child during the mother's absence, freely sharing accurate information even without being asked.

4) New models for acquisition of information are accompanied by new stresses

Certain changes in information transfer have already occurred. For example, the modern Yoruba child must look at, rather than away from, the parents while they talk in order to concentrate and pay attention. This is no longer considered rudeness.

Yet stress accompanies the emergence of new models due to links between information transfer, status, and social values. A focus group in the rural UNICEF project village of Olorunda in Oyo State, and interviews with project staff, revealed that illiterate parents experienced problems with the control of their school-going children, who ran off with and broke the toys provided by the project for preschoolers. The parents were operating on the traditional rule that once their children knew more than they did, they should not be controlled. Similar problems of lack of control over literate children have been reported to lead to refusal to farm, teenage pregnancy, and the like. Acquisition of information by juniors may be seen by elders as a threat to the settled social order.

Such concerns reach beyond Nigeria. In Kenya, a new boys' secondary school had a founding board of governors composed of respected local elders who had lacked the opportunity for secondary education. After two years of secondary education, the students began to disdain the directives of the board, remarking that they were only ignorant men. The relatively young headmaster had to use the authority which derived from his own university degree to endorse the authority of the much more senior governors, so as to render their management acceptable to the students. (Armstrong, personal communication)

Personal sense of entitlement to information was once determined by formal rank and was behaviourally reinforced by hierarchical interchanges. With the relative disempowerment of traditional hierarchies, this sense of entitlement appears to draw on new secular hierarchies, such as educational attainment, occupation and income, and on religious hierarchies. Statements of religious faith such as, "I am a child of God," may function as public assertions of the individual's sense of rank and entitlement to information and self-assertion.

When individuals no longer have a formally defined hierarchical niche, a nebulous sense of self-esteem appears to gain in importance.

Relatively lawless personalities who disregard social hierarchies may also achieve brilliantly where limited entitlement to information holds back their peers.

Rules of management of available resources

Payment for goods and services was traditionally based primarily on paying the provider with a fixed proportion of available resources, rather than with fixed quantities in kind or in cash on an item-by-item basis.

Community members of higher status were given priority in allocation of most resources. Seniors distributed the resources, operating under rules placing them under moral obligation to see that their juniors received portions that corresponded in size and quality to the rank of the junior member. During times of scarcity, this system continued to function even in the absence of surplus stocks for payment. No matter how scarce the resources, they could still be divided proportionally to the benefit of those responsible for provision and managing the system.

In modern economic systems, such in-kind transfers and rights of seniority now function in circumscribed domains that are secondary to, or in the service of, monetized economic power structures. Within the industrial power structure they may manifest as the legitimate symbols of power or, at the fringes, as quasi-legal or illegal means of biasing the established system. However, they remain at the core of the non-monetized domestic economic arrangements governing the nuclear family.

The implications for this manner of allocation of resources is that:

1) Limited commodities are rationed by seniority

The manner in which food and attention, stimulation, and information are distributed is central to the economic reward system that sustains production. In such a system, one would expect that the commodities functioning as the most basic symbols of reward would be those which would:

> make the distribution proportions consistently discernible, be frequently used and negotiated by everyone, and be in limited supply.

Food and information are in constant transaction. Food is absolutely limited by availability; information less so. Both are rationed in accord with seniority.

Family and community structure

The woman and her children

A mother and her children were the most elemental production unit in a family structure in which resources flowed from the children to both parents and from the wife to the shared polygamous unit governed by the father.

The concept of "housewife" familiar in the West was nonexistent in Africa. The wife was a farmer, a trader, a petty or sometimes a major producer of crafts or processed foods (e.g. among the Yoruba black soap or yam flour). The wife bore an extremely heavy load, although the load was possibly lighter among the Yoruba than among many other African ethnic groups in which women were also the primary agricultural producers. Among the Yoruba, men carried out most of the farming.

There was a concept of unlimited good in marriage and childbearing because every child and every wife was viewed as adding to the family's profits and prestige. Children were welcomed and loved with a hardy spirit of optimism. A woman's success was measured by her ability to bear children. A man had an equal need for children to carry on his lineage, which extended into the spiritual realm of the ancestors who continued to protect the living members of the family.

In the absence of a system in which wealth was based primarily on surpluses and had to be demonstrated in outward signs of material well-being, the cultural ideology viewed having extra wives and children as highly prestigious in and of itself. Whether in fact additional wives and children proved to be economically profitable or non-profitable, the rewards of prestige and social standing still accrued to the man for having wives and children and to the woman for having children. No material proof of profitability was required.

Wives required relatively little investment from husbands. Since the wife and her children would support themselves, there might be little perceived urgency for the man to plan for their support or to contribute materially to his wife's support. She was assumed to be self-sufficient.

Caldwell and Caldwell (1990) imply that communal land ownership and labour intensive traditional agriculture were part of a more general subsistence pattern that was universal in early farming communities prior to the accumulation of agricultural surplus. Within this pattern family structures tended to place a primary productive burden on the women. Yet the experience of African groups which have made the transition from hunting and gathering to settled agriculture since European penetration suggests that it may have been the cultural gender roles of pre-agricultural hunters and gatherers that placed responsibility on women for horticulture and hence agriculture.

Children also required relatively low levels of investment from their parents.

Children were below the mother in the proportional reward system described earlier. Mothers' concerns that the child should adapt to scarcity in this context would necessarily be less benign for the child than similar concerns in a system which favoured the child over the mother. In this system the youngest child must submit to greater deprivation than anyone else in the family once past early infancy.

It could be compassionate to keep the child relatively anesthetized to the transition, easing him or her as gently as possible from the favoured position of new infant to the very bottom of the hierarchy. Gentle means could include soothing rather than stimulating the child and not letting him or her taste certain delicacies of which the youngest would usually be deprived. In terms of stimulation, it might be better not to "wake up" the child through intensively active actions of any sort before he or she had survived transition through the period of lowest entitlement.

Attention rationing and food rationing within this structure were an adaptive response to the precariousness of the production system, and the limits of the mother's time and energy.

To the extent that men remain distanced from the immediacy of contemporary child-rearing expenses, they may hold onto a world view which justifies a belief that their wives' requests for support are excessive. Men who encounter economic difficulties may also increase rather than reduce their number of wives and children as an alternate source of self-esteem. Other cultural practices also heighten the necessity for multiple unions.

Shifts toward closer nuclear family ties are a recent phenomenon.

Couples who change to a closely bonded allegiance primarily to each other and to their nuclear family, a pattern noted among middle class Nigerian families by Caldwell (1977), may share a degree of economic security that women did not enjoy in earlier eras, and may be able jointly to allocate resources to their children in a qualitatively different manner. During the ethnographic study, four mothers of high scorers expressed satisfaction with the teamwork and cooperation they felt with their husbands in bringing up the children.

Postpartum taboo on sexual relations

Prohibition of sexual relations throughout the extended period of lactation usually lasting up to 3 years among the Yoruba and certain other groups formerly facilitated multiple unions and shaped the composition and age structure of the family workforce. Such postpartum taboos on sexual relations, believed to be universal in Africa in the pre-colonial era (LeVine *et al.*, 1990), were reinforced by the belief that semen entering the body during sexual relations poisoned the mother's milk. The institution of female circumcision may have made it easier for the woman to endure two to three years of sexual abstinence while she breastfed each child, and even to share a single room with her children for most of her life. Deprived of the new mother as a sexual partner, the husband was expected to turn his attentions to another wife.

The long birth interval and breast-feeding protected the child. It protected the nutrition and health of the last-born child, as well as increasing the attention which the mother could give him. This pattern is widely believed to be an adaptation that improved the rate of child survival where the post-weaning diet was low in protein.

However, prolonged breast-feeding, withholding of animal foods, and marginal malnutrition have also been suggested to strengthen the child's immunity to malaria (Lepowsky 1985). Writing about toddler malnutrition in the Vanatinai region of Papua New Guinea, Lepowsky quotes studies showing that the more poorly nourished individuals seemed more resistant to malaria or did not manifest as severe symptoms (Scrimshaw, Taylor and Gordon 1968, Beusel 1982, McGregor 1982, cited in Lepowsky 1985). She also cites studies indicating that a milk diet suppresses malaria infection, and that human infants on all-milk diets are known to be resistant to malaria (Maegraith *et al.*., 1952; Bray and Garnham, 1953; Maegraith, 1967, cited in Lepowsky, 1985).

Other researchers also have suggested, based on evidence from West Africa, that undernutrition protects children against lethal cerebral malaria (Hendrickse *et al.*., 1971; Edington, 1967). Quite apart from diet, however, the postpartum taboo might also help to protect a sleeping arrangement in which the mother could hold her sleeping cloth over the infant's body at night, in lieu of a mosquito net.

Household composition and age structure affected child tasks and training.

The age structure and composition of the traditional household played an important role both in determining expected labour contributions and in the training of children. A blueprint for labour expected from siblings and extended family members was set by the age composition and living arrangements of traditional families and communities. When the post-partum taboo guaranteed that all children were spaced about three years apart, with inevitable gaps caused by infant and child mortality, the ratio of adults to children and of older to younger children was relatively dependable.

The role of this expected birth succession in training groups of siblings to take on the tasks appropriate to their ages appears to be strong among the Yoruba and among the Kipsigis. It is commonly claimed among the Yoruba, that youngest children are spoiled, and that children of a previously barren woman or a woman whose previous children died in infancy are at risk of being spoiled. All of the same claims are also part of Zeitlin's German-immigrant American family heritage. Among the ten families studied ethnographically, one had an only child, who was perceived by a neighbour in the building to be spoiled for that reason.

Traditional living arrangements

Traditional housing and community structure facilitated the economic and social exchanges of productive labour and interactive support that sustained the family and the lineage. The traditional community was a stage set for its players, with numerous stage properties. Here all the various scenes of life could be played out according to known rules from day to day without fragmentation or disorientation.

The basic residential unit was a room shared by a mother and her children who lived with her until maturity. The larger domestic unit consisted of her husband, his other wives and their children, his elders, and other relatives. This larger unit incorporated the individual mother-child rooms into a compound with a yard in which cooking and child care were shared. The compound included separate rooms for adult males and a dormitory room for older boys. Compounds belonging to the same lineage would be clustered together in the same village or in the same urban neighbourhood.

1) Living together allowed mutual reinforcement by co-wives

The traditional compound accommodated polygamy in a manner which permitted co-wives to contribute to each other's prosperity. The compound gave each wife private living quarters in a shared courtyard. Although tensions could develop, shared food, cooking rotations, child care and other communal labour rewarded the co-operation of co-wives in traditional polygamous unions.

Competition between co-wives was minimized because traditional society emphasized group harmony and placed little value on conspicuous consumption of material goods. Each new wife increased the services available to the wives senior to her, and half-siblings contributed to each others' care. In a manner analogous to consumer goods, the presence of additional wives was a visible sign of wealth which increased the prestige of all household members.

2) The kinship group cared generally for preschool children

Multi-generational family units living in neighbourhoods densely populated by lineage members could rely on the community to supervise and socialize children from about the age of two or three. Little specific investment was needed in child care after the first two years of life, as the community supervisors of the children were family and lineage members who reaped benefits from the children's services directly as the children grew older. Given the similarity in family structure and the shared cultural background among neighbours, reciprocal child care services occurred naturally. The compound design provided a relatively safe enclosed play yard for the youngest children, within view of their caretakers.

It was traditional for relatives to provide periodic treats of food to the children of the compound, a welcome addition to the young child's diet given in an atmosphere of good cheer.

3) Leisure for interaction with children was available after dusk

In the absence of electricity, productive work usually came to a halt at dusk. In the dark by lamplight and moonlight, relatives and friends sat and enjoyed each other's company. This was a time for story telling, riddles, and singing as well as music and dancing on special occasions. Most compound members had leisure at this time to play with and educate children.

Chapter 4

Child care and rearing practices

Early precocity of African infants

Sub-Saharan African children have consistently been found to score significantly above North American and some European standards for child development on all indicators during the early months of life in more than a score of studies starting from the late 1950s (Durojaiye 1976; Gebber and Dean 1957; Goldberg 1970; Kilbride 1970; Liddicoat 1969; Munroe 1971a; Wober 1975, Chapter 1). African infants were generally reported to maintain their psychometric advantage into the second year of life or slightly beyond. Other studies comparing Caucasian and African children, particularly in South Africa, (where both sets of babies may have had African caretakers) found no differences. LeVine *et al.* (1990) question the validity of the earlier research studies, but concede that ages of crawling and walking are usually found to be earlier in African samples.

Agiobu-Kemmer, also found in a comparison between British and Nigerian infants aged from six to fifteen months (Agiobu-Kemmer 1984), that the Nigerian infants sat and crawled earlier than the British and were ahead of their British counterparts on most scales of the Piagetian infant assessment test designed by Uzgaris and Hunt (1975).

Physical contact, technical play and stimulation

Nigerian parents engaged their infants in social play and motor training for a greater percentage of the time, while British mothers spent more time involving their infants in technical play.

Whiten and Milner (1984) analysed information from the same children as Agiobu-Kemmer and observed that the Nigerian infants spent about twice as much time as the British in physical contact with a caretaker. However, the British infants were more frequently handled and positioned in a manner that enabled them to pay attention to the technical flexible manipulation of objects. British mothers scored three times higher than the Nigerians on a scale which measured the amount of time the caretaker spent structuring the infant's immediate posture and environment so that the child could manipulate and explore the uses and properties of objects.

LeVine and associates (1989) who compared behavioural data from 12 Gusii mother-infant pairs in Kenya with nine North American mothers and infants in an extensive longitudinal study also found that the African infants had more than twice as much physical contact with their caretakers than the Americans. They reported among the Gusii, however, what appear to be lower stimulation levels than among the Yoruba. The Gusii mothers were observed to avoid eye contact with their babies and systematically to calm them down when they were happy or excited, while the American mothers actively played with and stimulated theirs. American mothers were observed to spend more than twice as much time talking to their babies during the first ten months of life. Between one and two years, the Gusii child reached a low point in maternal attention since the mother generally was expecting a new birth while being very busy with economic activities. By the age of two years, he or she joined siblings and peers, and was supervised by the older children according to their age hierarchy.

The precocity in sensorimotor development widely reported for African children disappears in the second and third years of life. Studies of cognitive development in children aged from three to six years reveal this developmental trend. Yet because they become increasingly culture dependent, test scores for older children are difficult to evaluate.

Piagetian theory remains a major paradigm for understanding mental development at this age, and the basis for a large number of studies. Suchman (1966) found that on a sorting task, a sample of 120 Hausa children aged between three and five years preferred colour as the sorting criterion. His study concluded that shape had not emerged as a sorting criterion for these children.

Piagetian tasks

Piagetian cognitive type tests have shown the drop in precocity among

African pre-schoolers, their level of social development with regard to sibling and peer interactions is however quite good. There is however a heavy value placed on accurate recall and social development by the culture.

In a preliterate society, as Nigeria used to be, memory was a prized form of intelligence. For brain power, some children were given a powdered concoction called *isoye*, which would supplement the intelligence and assure a good memory.

Much of the Nigerian educational system, beginning with preschool lessons, continues to emphasize memorization and accurate recall of verbal information. Given the shortage of textbooks and inaccessibility of libraries, what children do not remember they cannot look up. Memorization continues to be valuable in the Nigerian context.

However, emphasis on rote memory may prove maladaptive to changing socioeconomic conditions, which reward a degree of flexibility and innovation. Additional emphasis on rearrangement and manipulation of what has been learned so as to apply it in new situations may prove important to children's cognitive development.

Conflict avoidance

Individual disregard of group norms in the older system threatened the survival of the family unit and of the community. Thus conflict avoidance and group harmony had higher priority than individual satisfaction and development. True sociality, which is committed to the support of all group members, and the ability to participate in the spiritual experience of oneness with the group are basic human values which characterize Africa (Setiloane, 1986).

The African seniority and support network tended to extend to relatively more distant family members than Asian or Eurasian kinship networks, in which support was more closely tied to the hereditary transfer of private property rather than lineage entitlement. Turnbull (1974) claims that the level of African production technology led to conditions in which such true sociality of the group was the only road to survival. African societies were therefore marked by cultural practices that functioned to avert conflict. Stealing within the kinship group blacklisted not only the thief but also his immediate relations, thus threatening to rupture their life support systems. Yoruba traditional child-rearing ethics were therefore very sensitive and strict with regard to stealing and to respect for seniority rights to material goods (Babatunde, 1987).

Implications for the allocation of food and information

1) Children were to be protected from what was perceived as temptation

Children often were not exposed to foods that might tempt them to steal or violate distribution norms. Some parents stated during focus groups that it was necessary for the children's moral training to prevent their exposure to coveted items, such as eggs and meat, which could motivate the desire to steal. Such protection may seek to preserve the innocence of childhood.

2) Social accountability was stressed

All goods entering and activities regarding the household were accounted for and confidentially managed according to the household seniority structure. Many of the spontaneous conversations between adults and children recorded in the ethnographic study consisted of the adult making sure that the child had respected the proper social rules and channels within the seniority system for reporting food and other items received, by reporting activities to the appropriate senior person, and by transferring physical objects to appropriate destinations. For example, one child given a ball by the project ethnographer was told to put it away until his father came home and could be informed.

These personalized confidential management rules could work efficiently with a group of limited size. However, they often required that action be put on hold in the physical absence of the senior decision maker.

3) Group sharing and group harmony were highly valued

Just as assembling around the family dinner table has been stressed in western tradition as an occasion for family bonding and communication, so eating from a common bowl has its lessons for Nigerian siblings. Children were supposed to experience group solidarity while practising the group's distribution rules peacefully. Parents in the ethnographic study tended to divide the food into pieces designated for each child but to leave the children to work out minor disputes on their own while eating. An adult might intervene periodically to teach manners and to settle major disputes, as did one child's lesson teacher who happened to be on hand when two sisters quarrelled over a piece of fish.

Urbanizing Yoruba siblings in our study, however, owned their own possessions, often including dishes, in contrast to siblings in some East African groups who are taught to share by not being encouraged to claim individual ownership of toys, dishes, or other objects.

4) Potentially divisive information was restricted

Information that might cause individuals to question the decisions of their superiors or cause conflict between peers was closely restricted. Conflict avoidance also extended to preventing spiritual or psychic mischief by creating extreme respect for the privacy of personal information that could cause envy or anger.

Actions that could be considered favouritism toward certain juniors by senior members are inherent in seniority structures. For the management structure, these are simply the measures through which they groom and train junior members according to their characteristics and capabilities. Senior members balance the ability of individual junior members against the requirements of the tasks to be performed in determining both task allocation and rewards.

Such treatment cannot be equal for all. Information regarding rewards to members of the group needs to remain confidential. Practices in modern corporations are parallel, as merit increases in salary for some but not for others cannot be publicized without disrupting working relationships. Where the production system is the microcosm of the extended family, the need for confidentiality about rewards may reinforce strict controls on information transfer to junior family members. In Nigeria and in other African countries, grandparents are known to set aside food or other rewards for favoured grandchildren, and give these secretly in order to avoid provoking jealousy.

Another reason for releasing information only on a need-to-know basis is a fundamental African perception that human beings are force fields (Setiloane, 1986) with the power to act invisibly (or perhaps subliminally) upon each other for good or evil, using personal information as a source of power for such action. Within the kinship group living and interacting in a confined geographical space, information was potentially inflammable and therefore tended to be closely guarded, particularly from children.

Challenges and resources for transition

1) Changes are resulting from schooling
Certain transitions have occurred spontaneously with the introduction of modern schooling. The school provides an objective evaluation of the child's abilities and performance and an external reward structure, embedded in an economic system in which the adult child no longer necessarily works for the family and therefore no longer depends on the fortunes of the extended family. By taking the tasks of selection, promotion and production out of the family, these changes ultimately remove the need for withholding food and information from the child in order to avert family conflict.

Conversely, these changes reward parents for feeding their children rich diets both of food and of information. However, it is extremely difficult to make such significant changes in values and practices, particularly when parents still need to rely in old age on traditional networks operating under the old rules of family sharing.

2) Conspicuous consumption has introduced new values
Urban families are exposed through billboards, radio and television to a culture of conspicuous consumption which competes with the traditional values of the seniority system. In focus groups in Makoko Lagos, parents expressed their pride in being able to buy fancy clothes for their young children, so that they could be seen to be keeping up with their neighbours.

For example, little girls might be dressed in relatively costly pink dresses. Yet these same parents still severely limited the amount of fish, meat and other foods they would give the girls in the interests of protecting their moral character.

(3) Solidarity with kinsfolk may produce conflict with the interests of the larger society.
Traditional socialization to respect the ownership of property has been claimed to extend only to the kinship group. The member of a kinship group who is a government functionary is not expected to steal from resources belonging to his own group, but he may be expected to take what belongs not to him but to the government, in order to service the needs of his kinship group (Ekeh, 1982). Even if he is caught, he tends to be approved by his kin as a good person.

Physical prowess

In previous times, economic production required physical dexterity, strength, and stamina, using technologies that were simple and labour intensive. In the absence of transport animals or wheeled vehicles, travel was on foot over many miles, and heavy loads were usually carried as head loads by human transporters. Agriculture using short handled hoes, scythes, and other iron instruments required strength and endurance. Tree crops were harvested by climbing.

Implications for the allocation of food and information

1) Motor development was an important objective of early child stimulation

High priority was placed on the infant's motor development, and traditional stimulation activities promoted early attainment of motor milestones. Rapid motor development could relate to survival skills requiring physical dexterity, and activities such as hunting, war and farming. Early walking made it possible for the child to accompany adults on foot and to start to learn to perform small tasks.

Focus groups with Yoruba mothers and grandmothers found a traditional preference for babies who were wiry and agile — children who learned to walk early without long remaining a burden to be carried. Walking was a major indicator of development. Folk wisdom relates that girls and later-born children walk earlier than boys and the first-born; and that spoiled children and children who are carried walk later. It is a disciplinary imperative for the child to begin to walk. The child was coaxed to start walking and was rewarded with singing and clapping. He might be given objects to hold so that he did not realize he was walking without support.

Caretakers also promoted early standing, sitting and crawling. Babies would be encouraged to stiffen their legs to support their weight from birth. From birth, infants were also carried upright on the back, usually supported by a cloth that needed to be frequently re-tucked (like a bath towel), entailing repeated moments during which the caretaker and infant co-ordinated their alignment and during which the infant was momentarily exposed to the freefall sensations of gravity. From the age of three months for girls and five for boys, babies were propped in a sitting position in a hole in the ground or with cushions. The later age for boys was out of fear of crushing the testicles.

Agiobu-Kemmer (1984) observed that the Yoruba mothers trained their infants to crawl by repeatedly placing objects just beyond their reach, while the Scottish mothers in her comparison study did not do so. She attributed the African children's precocity on Piagetian tests to the fact that their early mobility permitted them to explore spatial relationships and objects earlier and more actively than the British children. Yet the Yoruba mothers claimed in response to interview questions that they had done nothing special to train their children.

African mothers display fearlessness in promoting motor development which is not universally found. For example, the Positive Deviance Research Project in Indonesia found during focus groups with traditional midwives in Semarang, Central Java, that early sitting and standing was believed to damage weak ligaments and insufficiently hardened bones. In Java, where some infants were found to receive up to half their calories in rice from the first week of life onward, the local midwives reinforced a tradition that required the mother to hold the child in a horizontal position, forbidding the baby to be held upright against her shoulder until he had spontaneously attained a sitting position (Sockalingam *et al.*, 1990).

Traditional North American and European cultures of infant care also forbid placing infants in sitting or standing positions until they assume them spontaneously, for fear that the child's bones will bend. Endemic rickets in Europe in earlier centuries could have contributed to this cautious approach. Sub-Saharan African infants have generally been protected from this vitamin D deficiency disease, in which lack of exposure to sunlight causes inadequate calcification of the bones.

Archaeological and anthropological records suggest that African populations have experienced less severe cumulative young child malnutrition than populations descended from ancient agricultural and urban civilizations. Cohen (1990) reviewing prehistoric patterns of hunger describes a general pattern of decreasing diet quality and increasing morbidity and weaning-age malnutrition with each successive cultural transition from small bands of hunters and gatherers to intensive gatherers to settled farmers, and to the poor masses in urban civilizations. Descendants of such civilizations may typically have cultures of infant care that are adapted to fragile malnourished infants. This could explain positive African attitudes and high levels of skill with respect to stimulation toward early motor development milestones. Traditional African infant care skills should be treasured as a natural human resource, an adaptation producing optimal physical fitness that may otherwise have been lost to modern civilization.

2) Solid foods might be withheld until the baby walked

Heavy staple foods, such as cassava meal and pounded yam, tended to be withheld until the Yoruba child could walk, out of fear that he would become *wuwo*, a word applied to immobile older infants. This folk diagnosis of the "heavy or clumsy child" applied both to fat, normally nourished lazy babies and to malnourished, starch-fed babies with enlarged stomachs and marginal swelling from kwashiorkor.

Challenges and resources for transition

1) Changes in both child care and child accomplishments are inevitable

There is a need to avoid stereotyping which might classify one group as irrevocably advanced in one domain but delayed in another. However, child care practices and testable skill levels are not static, but rather in a state of inevitable and constant change.

Child care advice in the West has swung widely from one extreme to the other as populations struggle to adjust to changing conditions. Claims by some westerners that no one should intervene to suggest changes in developing country cultures may be inconsistent with the attitudes of these individuals toward progress in their home cultures.

The tests against which African infants were measured during the 1960s were based on norms derived from North American infants by Gesell during the 1930s (Gesell *et al.*, 1940). This was a time when U.S. paediatricians advised the mother to feed the infant only four hourly and to leave him lying in his crib or playpen most of the day. Mothers were not to indulge the child's desires to be held or fed, in order to avoid spoiling him. Extreme measures such as encasing the child's hands in mittens were also taken to prevent self-gratification by thumb sucking, for example. In the typical days described for infants and young children by Gesell and Ilg (1943) from infancy onwards the normative children spend most of their waking hours happily alone in their rooms, beds, carriages or play yards. It should be noted that a part of the rationale for rigidly scheduled infant feedings and for limitation of contact with the mother was to develop moral character.

2) *Some western customs may slow children's early development*

Modernizing Africans should be encouraged not to imitate negative practices from the industrialized nations which would inhibit their children's early development. In tests reported by Wober (1975) upper class African infants, who sometimes slept in cots and whose mothers had presumably been exposed to western child-rearing theories, scored lower on developmental tests in earlier months than the children of the poor, while tending to surpass poorer children after the first or second year of life. In Ile-Ife, Odebiyi (1985) found children of educated mothers more likely to be neglected than children of poorer mothers.

3) *African motor stimulation techniques deserve wider dissemination*

In-depth studies of traditional African stimulation of the very young child should be conducted to learn the interactions that promote early achievement of motor development milestones. Today's infants in industrialized countries are strong and well nourished and have no need to be treated as if they were fragile. Traditional infant massage should be included in this investigation.

4) *There is a need to give African parents access to child cognitive stimulation resources*

As parents traditionally invest in stimulating early motor development, they can be encouraged to expand this input toward stimulation of technical and cognitive skills. Children of all nationalities today face competition on the world market on account of globalisation; it is imperative to give African parents access to the child stimulation resources which they need to promote their children's technical skills.

For example, all of the children in the study played with objects such as sticks, balls, water, bottle caps, paper, and plastic containers. These toys, which promote imaginative and dramatic play, may need complementing by others which encourage perception of consistent relationships, precision of fit, and completion of a task. Sets of toys which fit together in a predictable way, such as nesting beakers or proportioned building bricks, illustrate principles of size, sequence, and relationship which more random play materials may not, thereby enriching both cognitive and manipulative skills.

The ethnographic study revealed dramatic differences in verbal interactions between low-scoring and high-scoring families. Both receptive and productive language skills of small children can receive increased stimulation and rewards without financial cost to the family.

Children's economic participation

Economic production relied on the contributions of children working with relatively low levels of adult supervision. Much has been written about the early start of productive labour in African as well as other traditional societies. In fact modern concepts of a prolonged childhood are recent. Under the guild system in medieval Europe, children assumed adult responsibilities at about the age of seven, when they could be apprenticed to work for their keep outside the home. Children were profitable to their parents. Agriculture, food processing, indigenous manufacturing and marketing were labour-intensive and there were many tasks that could be performed by children for the support of the family.

Surveys conducted by Caldwell (1977) indicated that Nigerian children began to contribute substantively to the family's subsistence by the age of five or six. The parents estimated that each child born would remit an amount of money to the parents equivalent to 10% of household income, in addition to providing old age and disaster security. Child care also was the work of children. In some African groups the job of nursemaid, given to girls of about seven to nine years, is formalized, with a special name (LeVine *et al.* 1990, Gabbidon 1991).

Traditional African culture trained children to be more responsible than modern Western children. Whiting and Whiting (1986) documented the greater social responsibility and maturity of East African Gusii children when compared to children of all other (non-African) culture groups in a six-country study. The greater responsibility of children in Africa still is beneficial to society. In general African youth are adequately socialized so that they are not unruly, or abusive toward their elders.

Implications for skills, information, and food distribution

1) Procedures and rules of conduct had to be simple
The need to rely on relatively unsupervised children required standardized procedures clear enough for children to carry out, and rules of conduct that were equally straightforward. All rules for supervision and conflict resolution had to be simple in order to function among the

very young, who rarely can make decisions based on logical operations.

The seniority system, applied among children, provided such a set of rules. The system orders that the older siblings command obedience from younger siblings and are responsible for the performance, conduct, and safety of the younger ones. Seniority in age might depend literally on date of birth so that a half-brother whose birth predated that of his half-sibling by only a few days would have seniority. Zeitlin observed two-to five-year-old Yoruba village children practising their mastery of the system by exercising their seniority rights to order one another to perform tasks during play, referring to adults to confirm the accuracy of their relative ages (Zeitlin, 1982). Zeitlin's two-and-a-half year old daughter, who lived with her in the village, soon mastered her own age-rank and the rules for her age.

2) Obedience to authority and behavioural conditioning were common teaching modes

Parents had to start early to teach skills and rules of conduct by conditioning rather than by application of logical reasoning. Behavioural conditioning and unquestioning obedience training were necessary because children responsible for serious work cannot be permitted to question authority and "play around" with procedures. Rules for food distribution also have to be clear and authoritarian in order to prevent the strongest from taking all.

Both the ethnographic study and focus groups with Lagos parents and grandparents revealed that many families' approach to preparing children to accept authority in times of scarcity was behavioural rather than through explanation and persuasion. They would restrict the child's food so that he would never get used to plenty, not developing expectations impossible to meet when times were hard.

One grandmother described her training of her grandchild through his school lunch money. One day she would give him one Naira (about US$ 0.10), the next day 30 kobo ($.03), the next 1.50 Naira, and so on, varying the amount randomly. She said that not being used to a fixed amount, he would never be able to accuse her of withholding money from him during hard times. By contrast, University of Lagos project team members asserted that they would use a more verbal and interactive style of teaching, explaining the concept of scarcity to their children and ask for their cooperation.

Challenges and resources for transition

Increasing technical complexity extends the duration of childhood by making it impossible for children to operate the mechanics of transport, production, service delivery, etc. A poignant example of a mismatch between traditional expectations and modern technology is an instance reported by Kranzler (1987), of a Samoan traditional healer who delegated the management required by the hospital for his daughter's juvenile diabetes to a 12-year-old sibling.

Unfortunately for stressed parents, the technical complexity of feeding and education of young children, according to modern standards of quality, is such that it cannot be left to sibling caretakers. Yet modernizing African parents still need the services of their children. Many parents are caught painfully between conflicting needs for their children to help them economically and simultaneously to excel in school. The style of parental attention and rewards that operate most effectively to train a young child to perform household chores differs from the style of interaction that trains him for good school performance and success in a modernized economy. Parental expectations of children are therefore undergoing modification.

Chapter 5

Nutrition among the Yoruba

Introduction

The distribution of nutritional characteristics in Nigeria follows the four dramatically different vegetational zones of the country and the agricultural activities in each of these regions. Protein deficiency, especially among young children, is a predominant problem in southern forest areas inland from the southern-most coastal belt of mangrove swamps and creeks (Atinmo, 1983; Adenike, 1988). This forest zone is the traditional home of the Yoruba ethnic group.

Generally, the northern Sahelian and savannah lands and the coastal parts of the country have fewer protein deficiency problems, as the environment allows for cattle rearing in the north, and for fishing along the coast. In the forest zone, the presence of the tsetse fly inhibits the raising of livestock, while game animals have become rare. The staples eaten in this region are yam and cassava which have particularly low protein content (Annegers, 1974; Ibukun-Olu, 1984).

Dietary intake

A high proportion of the Nigerian population has been estimated to have an inadequate dietary energy supply. Olayide (1978) computed average intake figures during 1971-1975 from estimated supplies of a wide variety of food commodities using a balance sheet approach. The average per capita daily intake of energy was 1980 kcal/day, about 83% of the minimum requirement recommended by FAO (1973). The per capita protein supply was then estimated at an ample 70 g/day, nearly two-thirds coming from sources other than animals and grain legumes. More recent figures document a situation in which per capita food supply has barely kept pace with population growth, food crops are sold for cash at prices unfavourable to producers, and disposable income for food has not kept up with sharp inflation.

As in many other developing countries, there is a marked inequality in income distribution and a steep gradient in nutrient consumption from the poorest to the wealthiest, with the result that a high proportion of the population has an intake of nutrients below requirements (Enwonwu, 1984). Yet, according to Enwonwu, misdistribution of protein foods within many Nigerian households is perhaps a more serious problem than the discrepancy in distribution of both protein and calories between the affluent and the poor groups.

Animal foods and moral degradation

Scarcity, cost, and ignorance of nutrient values are not the only factors in children's dietary intakes. Many researchers support Enwonwu's (1984) observation that

> In most ethnic groups in Nigeria, and even among the 'educated' the age-old system continues to allow a larger share of available nutrient-dense foods, including particularly foods of animal origin, to adult males than to children and women of childbearing age.

Food and feeding among the study sample were surrounded by moral sanctions. In repeated statements, mothers evaluated their children's social development by the child's ability to control appetite and to go without whining and begging for food. One two-year-old in the ethnography who repeatedly cried to be fed an hour or two after eating was the subject of ridicule in his family. The more general use of food for moral training applies to foods which may be plentiful in the family and for which the allocation does not emblematically reinforce the distribution function.

Fundamental habits of viewing eating in the context of character-building and self-discipline, and of achieving personal virtue by eating infrequent meals, may be reflected in the African practice of referring to meals by their staple component. This practice extends to a view that the staple is the food, whereas the stew ingredients such as fish, meat, vegetables, etc., are condiments or even luxuries without importance to the body. The Nigerian chooses whether to eat cassava or rice, not whether to eat meat or fish. Implicit in the way the choice is phrased is that the gratification expected from eating is experienced primarily in gradations of whole-body sensations linked to reduction of hunger and satisfaction of appetite, and secondarily in taste and aroma. It could be claimed that Yoruba cuisine, for example, makes finer distinctions between the textures and "weights" of its staple dishes than between the flavours of its stews.

Giving juniors a higher proportion also threatens the system.

Kolasa (1978), writing of practices restricting high status foods for children in Sierra Leone, suggests as a hypothesis that as food increases in availability with increasing wealth or decreasing prices, and males get all the food they desire, the strength of the belief or taboo against feeding children specific foods weakens. Kolasa (1978) and Cassidy (1980) also hypothesized that the withholding of meat and other high-quality foods is a response to potential food scarcity, designed to train the child to endure deprivation.

We believe that these explanations do not touch the root of the issue. We observed that parents are extremely reluctant to give more of symbolically important foods and of food in general to their young children out of fear that failure to train children to obey the proportional distribution rule may destroy the functioning of the management system, and hence the moral fabric of society. Such generosity with valued foods may also produce a socially unacceptable child.

For example, one grandmother in the Lagos low-income neighbourhood of Iwaya told the project team a cautionary tale of the troubles that had arisen when her son had married outside their ethnic group and the daughter-in-law had left him with their two young children. Her modern son had allowed these children to have as much food as they wanted, with the dire result that the children would steal meat from the family stew and take and misuse the property of others. One had even picked the lock on her door when she was out and had raided her house for food and money.

The belief that giving children more meat would be the beginning of the end and would ultimately lead them to steal was held by a large number of mothers in the study. This phenomenon has been widely reported from other countries of West Africa

Previous studies from Nigeria report that for preschool children, meat and eggs are restricted due to beliefs that too much of them cause the child's moral degradation (Ogbeide, 1974; Enwonwu, 1983; Ransome-Kuti, 1972, Vemury, 1978, Den Hartog, 1972). All these studies claim that such restriction contributes to the high malnutrition rate seen in Nigeria, although none has attempted precise measurement. Being predominantly concerned with nutrition, these writers have not explored the centrality of general food restriction, particularly of meat, in the moral training and socialization of the child.

Typical of such studies is Ogbeide's (1974) report of food taboos practised in former Midwest Nigeria (now Edo and Delta States), most having to do with foods of animal origin. In most parts of the state, meat and eggs were not given to children because parents believed these foods would make the children steal. Onuoha (1980) stated that it was considered most uneconomical to eat an egg that could produce a chicken, which would in turn fetch money when sold. The most senior males in the family were the only ones allowed to cook and eat the eggs unhatched by the hens. "Children were completely forbidden to eat eggs for fear that they might develop 'sweet tooth' which would lead them to steal when they grew up" (Onuoha, 1980).

Similarly Osuhor and Etta (1979) reported from Zaria, Northern Nigeria, that the low consumption of protein due to taboos and prohibitions of meat and eggs to infants and toddlers were contributory factors in protein energy malnutrition among the children attending an under-fives clinic. Cherian (1985) in her report of infant feeding attitudes and practices in Zaria related that egg is often not given because of the belief that small children, having developed a taste for this purchased food, may steal eggs from rich homes which regularly buy them.

Of interest is the fact that fish, which was the most frequent animal food for the Lagos State children of the present study, is not claimed to compromise the child's character. Yet, the ethnographic study determined that fish was rationed to the children like meat, in the same very small slivers compared to the size of the mother's portion. Fish and meat are categorized together by some parents in a belief that they may cause worms.

Although there is a broad literature concerning withholding of animal foods, no studies were found regarding the practice of rationing of staple foods. It is unlikely that routine rationing practices would give rise to cultural prohibitions or taboos.

A survey was carried out by Onuoha (1980) to determine the nature and extent of prevailing food habits and beliefs among the Ibo in south-eastern Nigeria. Thirteen food items, including some that were known not to be subjects of any taboos, were drawn up and 1506 people of both sexes from one community were selected and interviewed on their food habits and beliefs. It was found, generally, that staple foods such as yams, cassava and *garri* (cassava meal), and beans did not have taboos against them while high-protein animal foods like egg, beef or local cows' meat, pork, antelope meat, fresh fish, and snails were prohibited by one subgroup or another. The Yoruba have similar food taboos which interestingly also include vegetables like okra (okro).

Nutritional status of children under five

A nationally representative survey conducted by the Institute for Resource Development (Maryland, USA) with the Federal Office of Statistics (Lagos) produced a report with data showing children's nutritional status. Information was collected from 8,781 women aged 15-49 and 8,113 children aged 0-5 years. Table 5.1 shows the percentage of children under five years of age classified as undernourished according to height-for-age, weight-for-height, and weight for age indices, by age and some demographic traits. Nationally 45% of the children are stunted, with 22% being severely so while only 9% are wasted. Stunting increases with age up to about 12 years of age and also when birth intervals are shorter than 24 months. The South West region corresponding roughly to Yoruba speaking Nigeria has the lowest percentages for stunting and wasting.

Gurney and Omololu (1971) conducted a nutritional survey in two villages of Southwestern Nigeria. The anthropometric results of their study showed that the failure of growth seemed to affect the weights and heights of the children between one and five years equally with respect to percentages of children below 80% of weight-for-age and 90% of height-for-age. In children under 12 months of age, 28% were below 80% of standard weight, while 3% were below 90% of standard height. Recent data from a two-year study of more than 300 rural Yoruba children from Kwara State (Guptill *et al.* 1989) reveal more severe malnutrition among children in the first three years. The level of stunting (height-for-age Z-score <-2 SD) in these children increased steadily from less than 5% in the 0-2 month age group, to 20% at 9-14 months, over 30% at 21-23 months, and just below 70% at 33-35 months. This study found that delayed introduction of solid foods is a common practice, and that by 12 months fewer than half of the children had had solid foods introduced into their diets. The level of wasting (weight-for-height Z-score <-2 SD) increased from about 5% in the 0-2 month age group, reached its peak at about 25% in the 9-11 month age group, and decreased steadily to less than 5% in the 33-35 month age group.

Table 5.1: Nutritional status by socioeconomic characteristics

Percentage of children under fives who are classified as undernourished according to three anthropometric indices of nutritional status: height-for-age, weight-for-height and weight-for-age, by selected socio-economic characteristics, Nigeria 1990

Socio-economic characteristic	Height-for-age		Weight-for-height		Weight-for-age		
	% below −3SD	% below −2SD[1]	% below −3SD	% below −2SD[1]	% below −3SD	% below −2SD[1]	Number of children
Residence							
Urban	13.7	35.0	1.5	7.2	6.8	26.3	1,278
Rural	24.7	45.5	1.8	9.6	13.5	38.5	4,287
Region							
Northeast	30.1	51.9	3.2	11.3	18.6	44.6	1,199
Northwest	28.8	50.4	2.7	12.1	14.2	43.8	1,351
Southeast	17.1	36.6	0.6	7.6	9.5	29.6	1,893
Southwest	14.3	35.6	0.9	5.5	6.3	26.9	1,122
Mother's education							
No education	26.3	48.1	2.2	11.0	14.9	41.2	3,283
Some primary	17.5	38.6	0.9	8.2	9.6	31.4	618
Completed primary	18.9	39.7	1.5	5.8	8.5	29.8	899
Some secondary	15.3	35.9	1.0	5.8	7.0	28.4	347
Completed secondary/higher	9.3	23.1	0.9	4.6	3.9	17.4	415
All children	22.2	43.1	1.8	9.1	12.0	35.7	5,565

This pattern of high wasting followed by high stunting suggests a problem first of food energy and later of food quality as well. Between the ages of 9-11 months, the rural children were not getting enough to eat, probably because breast milk alone was not sufficient for their growth and the liquid maize pap used to supplement breast milk was very low in nutrient density.

By the time the children were 24-36 months old, they received proportionately more calories, but by this time deficiencies in the quality of the weaning diet were also evident in the rapidly increasing prevalence of stunting.

Deterioration of nutritional conditions

The degree of stunting particularly among low-income children has increased significantly over the past 30 years. Gurney and Omololu's sample of rural children of 20 years ago also were significantly less stunted than the Kwara State children of 1989. This deterioration may be attributed to the overall decrease in per capita food availability noted above, resulting in part from structural adjustment programmes (referred to in Nigeria as the SAP). The increase in stunting may also be attributed to increased reliance on cassava as the staple food of the poor (Annegers, 1973).

As in many developing countries, starchy staples make a large contribution to the total energy value of most diets in Nigeria. The major staple foods used vary greatly in their protein content. The percent of calories derived from protein in these staples ranges from less than 1% in cassava to 11% in sorghum and millet (Annegers, 1973).

The various starchy staples are used in distinct areas of the country as a result of crop ecology, historical diffusion, storage properties, and yields within the varying climatic zones of Nigeria. Cassava originated in South America and was diffused across the continent of Africa from South America and Asia (Idusogie, 1982; Annegers, 1973). Idusogie (1982) has observed that many elderly people in predominantly root-eating Nigerian communities are not used to eating cassava products because cassava was not grown or used as food in their childhoods. This suggests that cassava was perhaps introduced into Nigeria late in the nineteenth century.

Cassava has now become ubiquitous and a popular staple in many parts of the country, the food crop giving the highest calorie yield per hectare in Nigeria. The Federal Government of Nigeria and UNICEF estimate that with present day yields, a farmer needs to plant at least three-quarters of a hectare with cassava to feed an average family, but would need to plant much more of any other staple crop. Since more than half of the farms consist of one hectare or less, most rural households cannot now produce enough staple foods to meet their calorie requirements, and are forced to rely heavily on cassava. With a current population growth rate estimated at 3.2%, this situation is not improving.

Cassava is easy to plant, repels pests and is tolerant of a wide range of growing conditions, so that it can be grown in all the climatic zones of Nigeria except the Sahel. Cassava can be grown on poorer soils, or at the end of rotation cycles after maize, yams, or rice have depleted the soil.

Although most varieties need to be fermented during processing in order to remove hydrocyanic acid, the cassava meal which is the usual end product of fermentation, grating, and oil-free frying of the grated granules, has the advantage of being a convenience food which can be stored almost indefinitely and instantly reconstituted into a gel with boiling water, drunk in granule form with cold water, or eaten dry with palm oil.

Figures 5.1 and 5.2 show the per cent of a two-year-old child's protein requirement obtained from 800 kcal of grains, most roots, tubers, fruits, and cassava, and the increase in requirements for high-quality protein foods when cassava replaces traditional southern Nigerian staples. Table 5.1 shows the foods and nutrient values summarized in the figures.

It is evident from these computations that traditional indigenous grains of West Africa provide a basic minimum of protein for the young child with little complements from high-quality protein foods. Traditional starchy roots and plantain require somewhat more complements. However, cassava is so low in protein that it demands unrealistic quantities of high-protein foods, e.g. more than three ounces per day of meat, or ten ounces of cow-peas, if the child is to attain a safe level of protein intake set by FAO, WHO, and UNU (WHO 1985). Therefore increased reliance on cassava tends to lead to deterioration in diet quality.

Religious symbolism and sacrament with regard to food

Food had religious symbolism derived from rituals that extended the distribution and management rules of the human seniority hierarchy into the realm of the divine. The extension of the kinship seniority system beyond the grave into this realm has important implications for the distribution of food. Divine beings and ancestors are most senior in the system. Heads of lineage and heads of families are their representatives on earth.

The routine ritual sacrifices of traditional Yoruba religion rely on animals, birds, and fish to propitiate the "unseen mouths," of those above. Each of these foods may have symbolic significance in folk perceptions that correspond to their significance in such sacrifices, e.g. chickens to ward off death (as in the European folk belief that the spirits return to the grave at the cock's crow), or fish, which act as messengers to the divine by seeking out spirits wherever they may reside in the waters. This fact may lend animal foods special resonance even for the majority who now belong to the world religions of Christianity and Islam (Chief Atanda, personal communication).

Table 5.2: Adequacy of various African staples in meeting the protein requirement (RQ) for two-year-old child[1]

Met by (%)	Calories from protein[2] in staple (%)	Protein[3] in 800kcal of staple (gm)	Percent of child's protein RQ 800kcal of staple
Grains[4]			
Rice (brown or hulled)	9%	10.9	70%
Sorghum (average of all varieties)	12%	14.8	95%
Millet (African)	9%	10.9	70%
Wheat (Flour)	15%	17.8	115%
Maize (native ground)	11%	12.5	81%
Grains including wheat	11%	13.4	86%
Grains excluding wheat	10%	12.3	79%
Starchy roots, rubbers, fruits	6%	7.3	47%
Yam and potato	7%	8.6	56%
Yam (African)	6%	7.6	49%
Taro (cocoyam)	7%	8.4	54%
White potato	8%	9.9	64%
Plantain and sweet potato	4%	5.3	34%
Plantain	4%	4.2	27%
Sweet potato	5%	6.3	41%
Cassava	1%	1.5	10%
Meal (gari)	1%	1.5	9%
Flour (lafun)	1%	1.6	11%

---

[1] Zeitlin, M. F. and L. V. Brown, "Household Nutrition Security: A Development Dilemma," Consultant Report to Food and Agriculture Organization (FAO), 1991.

[2] Raw protein values used in assuming 1gm protein = 4 kcal energy

[3] Protein figure adjusted for quality assuming 85% diet digestibility, 70% amino acid score.

[4] Values are for uncooked staples due to variations in nutrients by varying cooking methods.

Bascom (1949) reported that meat was a food for ceremonies and special occasions, and only the chiefs and wealthy could afford to buy it regularly in the market or to kill a domestic animal simply for food. According to Bascom, British foreign influence increased the amount of meat in the average Yoruba diet even though meat was still considered a prestige food.

In addition to fears regarding spoiling and scarcity, there are published studies from various parts of Africa regarding the religious significance of food as an expression of totemic or other spiritual relationships which may manifest in different needs and restrictions for different individuals. While related to seniority, these spiritual concerns extend and transcend it. These factors have been judged to influence the distribution of food among members of the same family (Enwonwu, 1984; Nutrition Economics Group, 1984; Van Esterik, 1984).

Chief Atanda, Secretary of the Yoruba Ifa Traditional Healing Association (1989) in an interview has explained that in earlier days, because meat was obtained by hunting which involved a risk, a ritual was established whereby the oldest person was given the largest share. Meat was not regarded as part of essential foods; it was special. Its distribution reflected that value, the biggest share going to the head of the household who presumably protected the household and was the one taking the risk of hunting for the meat. Even today, when people do not literally go off to hunt for meat in order to live, this symbolic ritual persists in family food sharing patterns.

The rejection of eggs and chickens as food by certain members of the community is especially widespread in Africa. According to Simons (1961), this may have arisen out of the belief that eating these foods will bring about human infertility. Eggs are often regarded as symbols of fertility, so playing a role in magical and ceremonial life on occasion. Eggs could be eaten on rare occasions when a traditional doctor prescribed them as one of the ingredients in a medicinal concoction.

Implications for food distribution

The intra household distribution of animal foods, particularly of meat, had sacramental overtones.

Traditionally, the slaughter of a domestic animal always was conducted as a sacrifice preceded by prayers to ancestors or other divinities who were offered the blood. After the various blessings, the best portions would be offered to the adult male head of household, who was the living representative of the divine authority protecting the lineage and the family. It was then the father's role to apportion the meat to the rest of the family, reserving for himself the largest and best pieces. Feelings about the special entitlement of the father to meat were found to run deep even among Christian focus group members, and are a common theme emerging from the focus groups and the ethnographic study.

Under specific conditions adult males might feel motivated to redistribute foods

Traditionalists agree that the sacramental overtones of the male entitlement to receive and divide high-quality animal foods are the grounds through which the father can be motivated to reapportion meat or fish to meet the nutritional needs of the younger children. Having received this food as his right, the traditional system of responsibility requires him to share it out for the best use of the family. According to this theory, his obligation to put the well-being of the kin group (his family) first holds, even if this means that he must change for these particular foods the proportional allocation noted above as the basis of rewards under the seniority system.

Both the ethnographic study and focus groups repeatedly uncovered a pattern by which fathers already had the right to "spoil the child with meat." The mother might give the child his strictly limited share, and then if the father were available and favourably disposed towards the child, the child would eat again with the father. At that time the father would give the child additional meat and fish from his portion. The mothers' official attitude towards this practice was that they disapproved of such spoiling but that it was the father's right to do so. Yet the tones in which the mothers pronounced this attitude tended to express veiled pride in having a husband who took such care of the child.

Challenges and resources for development

Nutrition messages and interventions require sensitive pre-testing

As food distribution is integral to seniority systems, customary resource allocation, moral training, and conflict avoidance, as well as religious tradition, an unadorned message to mothers to give more animal food to the young child encounters formidable barriers. It may not even be perceived as a rational communication.

Yet the message to increase the child's protein foods along with other foods was felt to be vital for the following reasons:

Most children received only a fraction of their daily (FAO/WHO/UNU, 1985) protein requirements.

A noticeable cause for this shortfall, observed in the ethnographic study, was that the mothers as well as the fathers ate generous portions, particularly of fish, but very strictly limited the fragments given to the young children.

Good manners required that protein-rich foods be eaten last after finishing an accompanying portion of staple foods. Therefore increase in the protein food component of the diet implied an increase in overall food quantity.

A community-based intervention was undertaken in which community workers first detected nutritional stunting of the children using the tallstick (Zeitlin *et al.*, 1990). This alerted the mother to the existence of a problem. The community workers then presented a scientific distribution rule promised to potentially improve the child's school prospects, and this idea did seem to be well accepted.

Ways of involving the father through his traditional role still should be investigated

Our study population had two styles of meat apportionment. The more traditional style gave the entire amount to the father and awaited his distribution. The more modern and universally practised style provided for different cooking and eating times and for purchase from vendors. The mother apportioned the pieces according to the family's distribution rules, still giving the father the largest share, which he in turn could share with the children. In the case of fish, which was eaten almost daily, apportioning by the mother was the expected form of distribution.

Some focus group members believed that reallocation of a scarce amount of meat or fish could best occur if the father, mother, and child all ate together, in which case both the father and the mother could quietly favour the child if they understood that this food was needed for the child's development. The suggestion that father, mother and child eat together would appear to combine the presentation of the meat to the father according to traditional entitlement with modern nuclear family values of companionship.

Many fathers in the ethnographic study took the role of provider of snacks and treats. These might occasionally be barbecued beef (*suya*) but typically were sweets, sodas, and biscuits rather than more nutritionally valuable foods such as *akara*. Encouraging fathers to bring home higher-protein snacks might be linked to their traditional roles as distributors of protein foods. It would be useful to pursue these questions and those discussed by Ojofeitimi (1984) in search of educational messages.

Alternative moral training methods can be encouraged
Food almost always provides the occasion for parents to train and discipline their children; its withholding is not the only option. Parents also train with food by insisting that the children eat whatever nourishing foods have been prepared whether they enjoy them or not.

Attention, social approval, and control of time also are available to inculcate proportional distribution functions, and for child training. Among middle class Nigerian parents who have the resources to do so, there appears to be a trend towards disciplining the child through control of time and place — play time, study time, bedtime, etc. — which takes the place of the use of food. However, control of the child's time is problematic in crowded housing conditions in which five or more persons may share a room, so that, for example, the child cannot be put to bed at a set time.

Withdrawal of attention from the child as a form of discipline is considered inhumane among the Yoruba. Disciplining the child through social disapproval, using laughter and ridicule, is found among other peoples in Africa and Asia but is relatively less common among the Yoruba.

The project's community-based workers encouraged mothers to discipline their children "with the stick" if they disobeyed and also to teach them proper social conduct verbally. Focus groups and semi-structured interviews both with academics and with traditional opinion leaders reached consensus that this stepped-up verbal teaching and modelling of conduct combined with firm discipline could, at least on the surface, replace the use of food in child training. Changes in discipline accompany more fundamental shifts in parent-child interaction and in the concept of the family.

Reference to school success removes food and information from the domain of traditional proportional distribution
The community-based workers, in teaching mothers to increase the child's number of servings of protein foods per day to meet WHO/FAO/UNU requirements, appealed to the parents' desire for their children to perform well in school. In fact, parents appeared to be

receptive to change with school as the rationale, tending to view school achievement as leading to job success for the child. Reference to the school system, the new legitimizing hierarchy, removes the issues of feeding and stimulation from the rules embodied in the traditional hierarchy.

Section III

The field report

Chapter 6

Socio-economic and demographic characteristics of study sample

Positive deviance studies attempt to recruit uniformly low-income samples in order to identify income-independent factors that distinguish between more and less adequate coping with the stresses of child rearing under conditions of poverty. In this case low-income neighbourhoods were sought, and families living in high-quality houses were deliberately excluded. Nevertheless the sample varied socio-economically and this variability was of interest to both the primary and the cultural distance hypotheses of the study.

This section describes the socio-demographic and economic characteristics of the sample. Under each subheading, we first describe the sample by rural-urban location, presenting data only from the systematic sample. We then inspect characteristics that differ by child development group including children from both the systematic sample and the purposive malnourished sample. The small rural sample was included in this contrast because much preliminary analysis provided evidence that the basic relationships between variables were the same in the three locations. On variable after variable, differences between the locations appeared to fall along the same continuum, representing differences in degree rather than differences in kind.

Table 6.1 summarizes housing conditions and source of water by location, while Table 6.2 presents an overview of the socio-demographic characteristics of the systematic sample (excluding the purposive malnourished sub-sample). According to the sample selection procedures described earlier, 11% were rural, 41% semi-rural and 48% urban. Although compounds represent the traditional Yoruba housing type, fewer than 10% of the families lived in traditional compounds. Ninety percent of the rural to 67% of the urban lived in face-to-face housing, the modern variant of traditional compounds. Out of this 71% of households lived in a single room, with overall averages of 5.5 persons per household eating from the same pot and 3.6 persons per room.

Table 6.1: Housing conditions and water supply by location

	Rural (N=20)	Semi-rural (N=74)	Urban (N=86)	Total (N=180)
Housing type				
Face-to-face	90%	79%	67%	74%
Compound or flat	10%	8%	10%	9%
Detached	0%	15%	24%	17%
Wall construction				
Mud	65%	14%	0%	13%
Corrugated iron	0%	3%	15%	9%
Cement blocks	35%	83%	85%	79%
Roof construction				
Thatched	15%	0%	0%	2%
Asbestos sheets	20%	32%	35%	32%
Corrugated iron	65%	67%	64%	65%
Concrete	0%	1%	1%	1%
Floor construction				
Mud	5%	3%	0%	2%
Wood	5%	0%	2%	2%
Cement	90%	90%	69%	80%
Linoleum	0%	7%	27%	16%
Tiles	0%	0%	1%	1%
Physical condition of the house				
Very poor	10%	9%	16%	12%
In need of repairs	65%	39%	56%	51%
In good condition	20%	51%	24%	34%
New paint or furniture	5%	1%	4%	3%
Electricity in house	10%	66%	98%	75%
Source of water				
Stream	74%	1%	1%	9%
Well	5%	19%	1%	9%
Rainwater or tank	0%	13%	1%	6%
Borehole	5%	28%	0%	12%
Tap	16%	39%	96%	64%

Table 6.2: Socio-demographic characteristics by location

Means (SD) and percents

	Rural (N=20)	Semi-rural (N=74)	Urban (N=86)	Total (N=180)
Number of rooms	1.3(0.5)	1.5(0.8)	1.4(0.8)	1.4(0.8)
One	70%	70%	72%	71%
Two	30%	17%	17%	19%
Three to four	0%	12%	10%	10%
Household size	4.5(1.5)	5.6(2.4)	5.6(2.3)	5.5(2.3)
Persons per room	3.2(7.6)	3.6(6.7)	3.8(7.1)	3.6(7.1)
Age of mother	28.6(8.6)	27.9(5.8)	28.7(5.5)	28.4(6.0)
Mother's number of children	3.2(1.6)	3.1(1.7)	3.4(1.7)	3.3(1.7)
Percent of mothers earning income	100%	98%	99%	99%
Percent working away from home	63%	69%	58%	63%
Mother's years of education	5.9(3.5)	6.4(4.0)	7.3(3.5)	6.8(3.8)
Percent polygamous unions	89%	47%	33%	45%
Mother's religion				
Muslim	30%	43%	39%	40%
Roman Catholic	15%	3%	1%	3%
Indigenous Protestant	45%	39%	51%	45%
Foreign Protestant	0%	14%	18%	10%
Traditional	10%	1%	0%	2%
Other	0%	0%	1%	0%

Mothers were on average 28.4 years old, had 4.3 years of schooling and 3.3 children. Almost all, 99%, worked for income, with 63% working at a distance from home at least part-time. Fathers had on average 6.8 years of schooling, 4.7 children and often more than one wife. The percentage of polygamous unions decreased from 89% in the rural to 33% in the urban sample. It would appear that modernization tended to erode polygamy.

Fifty-eight percent of the mothers were Christians, and 40% Muslims. Ten percent of the rural but none of the urban mothers claimed to practise traditional Yoruba religion. Of the Christians, 78% belonged to the relatively new Nigerian Christian sects drawing membership from the older Protestant and Catholic denominations. 17% belonged to foreign Protestant denominations and 5% to the Roman Catholic Church.

A variety of socio-economic factors have been associated with child growth (Zeitlin, Ghassemi and Mansour 1990). Those which were investigated in this study included parental education and media exposure, occupation, food expenditure by source, maternal income and the child care assistance available to mother.

Education, literacy and media exposure

Table 6.3 displays parental education and mother's literacy, revealing a population that has made significant investments in education for at least two generations and that appears to have consistently favoured boys' over girls' schooling. Overall 45% of the mothers' fathers and 19% of their mothers had attended school. In the present generation, fathers had on average from six to seven years of education, and only 10% had no schooling contrasted to 30% who had completed secondary or had some post-secondary schooling. Mothers averaged 4.3 years, with 35% unschooled and only 11% who had completed secondary school. The rural-urban difference in schooling appeared greater for women than for men. In the small rural sample 47% of the women, but none of the men, had never attended school.

More than half of the mothers could read Yoruba, more than a third English and 7% Arabic. Overall 57% claimed reading skills in at least one language. Education differed by religion, however, with 55% of Muslim versus 74% of Christian mothers; and 83% versus 93% of fathers having attended school. The difference in boys' education by religion was apparent in the mother's fathers' generation in which 54% of Christian versus 36% of Muslim fathers had attended school. Of the sample mothers, 47% of Christians versus 26% of Muslims could read English; 69% versus 30% could read Yoruba; and 68% versus 45% were literate in any language. By contrast 17% of Muslim and 3% of Christian mothers could read Arabic.

An additional measure of the mother's ongoing education and exposure to current events was her ability to name states of Nigeria, radio and TV programmes (Table 6.4). Of interest is the ability of three-fourths of the mothers to name four or more states, and the fact that the women knew on average twice as many TV as radio shows by name. It is worthy of note that Western Nigeria has had the longest Radio and Television broadcasts in the indigenous language of the area – Yoruba. This is likely the source of this impressive knowledge of current affairs.

Table 6.3: Mother's and father's education, mother's literacy and maternal grandparents' education by location

Means (SD) and percents

	Rural (N=20)	Semi-rural (N=74)	Urban (N=86)	Total (N=180)
Last year of school completed by mother	2.2(2.5)	4.2(3.8)	4.8(3.8)	4.3(3.8)
No formal education	47%	37%	29%	35%
Some primary	26%	18%	13%	17%
Primary completed	26%	24%	29%	27%
Some secondary	0%	8%	16%	11%
Secondary completed	0%	13%	12%	11%
Last year of school completed by father	5.9(3.5)	6.2(3.9)	7.3(3.6)	6.7(3.7)
No formal education	0%	17%	7%	10%
Some primary	35%	11%	17%	17%
Primary completed	50%	34%	31%	34%
Some secondary	5%	23%	31%	25%
Secondary completed	10%	3%	6%	5%
Literacy of mother				
Reads Yoruba	15%	55%	67%	56%
Reads English	5%	34%	47%	37%
Reads Arabic	5%	5%	8%	7%
Grandparents education				
Mother's mother went to school	15%	14%	24%	19%
Mother's father went to school	40%	35%	58%	45%

Parental occupation

Table 6.5 shows the occupations of both parents. Although 5% of women originally claimed to be unemployed housewives, only 1% did not report either personal income or personal contribution to food expenditure. The majority of mothers were either petty vendors selling from home or petty traders, ranging from 67% in the urban to 80% in the semi-rural area. Higher occupational categories, from skilled labourer to professional, comprised 20% among the urban, 7% in the semi-rural and 10% of the rural sample. Middle-level market women and farm labourers totalled 10% of the rural but only 1-2% in the other two sub-samples.

According to the traditional Yoruba pattern, rural vendors whose husbands were farmers were more likely to be marketing the farm products through a concessionary purchase arrangement. Therefore, they tended to be substantial rather than petty vendors, even when they sold from home.

Table 6.4: Mother's exposure and general knowledge by location

Percents

	Rural (N=20)	Semi-rural (N=74)	Urban (N=86)	Total (N=180)
Number of states in Nigeria currently identified:				
None	1.1(0.8)	1.8(0.4)	1.8(0.4)	1.7(0.5)
One to three	26%	0%	1%	4%
Four or more	37%	76%	82%	74%
Names of radio programmes identified:	0.7(0.8)	0.9(0.8)	1.0(1.0)	1.0(0.9)
None	47%	33%	36%	36%
One to two	47%	44%	29%	38%
Three	0%	21%	26%	21%
Four or more	7%	2%	9%	6%
Number of TV programmes identified:	1.1(1.1)	1.7(0.9)	2.3(0.8)	1.9(1.0)
None	40%	13%	7%	13%
One to two	20%	23%	3%	13%
Three	27%	46%	47%	45%
Four or more	13%	18%	43%	30%
Media and education exposure scale	7.6(4.8)	12.9(7.7)	16.2(7.7)	13.9(7.8)

Trading is a Yoruba way of life. Petty vending is a less serious form of trade engaged in by young girls learning to sell, less astute business women, older women, and women who have other reasons not to engage in major commercial activities. While the Yoruba have traditionally moved raw materials between farms and urban markets, the semi-rural settlements are a new phenomenon. Semi-rural women are less likely to be geographically positioned for major commerce since they are distanced both from the raw materials and the markets. Their vending patterns may therefore be more likely to remain at the petty trade level, insuring that every woman has some income to call her own, no matter how little, but also leaving women more dependent on their husbands' incomes.

Although being a housewife involved exclusively in domestic rather than productive labour is not a part of traditional African culture, this concept appears to have emerged as an alternative for a few women. Two of the mothers of high scoring children in the ethnographic study noted with apparent pride that they would not have to work for money, but that they did so only "to help out". Recent curtailment of women's independent income-generating capacity, with the predominance of private land ownership since the 1960s and the distance of semi-rural women from either farm production or major urban markets, could also influence such a shift.

Table 6.5: Mother's and father's occupations by location

Percents

	Rural (N=20)	Semi-rural (N=74)	Urban (N=86)	Total (N=180)
Mother's occupation:				
Housewife earning no income	0%	2%	1%	1%
Petty vendor selling from home	55%	36%	42%	40%
Low-level market woman	25%	54%	25%	36%
Medium-level market woman or labourer	10%	1%	2%	2%
Skilled labourer or craftswoman	5%	4%	16%	11%
Clerical worker	0%	1%	6%	3%
Higher-level shopkeeper/owner	5%	2%	4%	3%
Professional	0%	0%	4%	2%
Father's occupation:				
Unskilled labourer	11%	0%	1%	2%
Farmer or fisherman	53%	19%	9%	18%
Low-level vendor	0%	10%	2%	5%
Skilled labourer	16%	38%	46%	39%
Taxi driver	11%	11%	11%	11%
Clerical worker	5%	7%	15%	10%
Clergyman, Imam or Ifa priest	5%	1%	9%	5%
Higher-level shopkeeper or businessman	0%	4%	2%	2%
Professional	0%	10%	5%	6%

The largest occupational categories for the fathers were skilled labour in the urban (46%) and semi-rural (38%) samples, and farmer/fisherman (53%) in the rural. Taxi drivers made up 11% in each group. Higher-level occupations such as clerical, business, or professional were 22% in the urban, 21% in the semi-urban and 5% in the rural groups. Unskilled labour was substantially represented only in the rural group (11%). Unskilled urban labourers would have been found in the various peri-urban neighbourhoods with high proportions of rural-to-urban in-migrants, particularly from other parts of the country. Of the urban fathers 79% fell into the skilled labour, taxi driver, or higher occupational categories, versus 70% of the semi-rural and 32% of the rural fathers. Clergymen as a group were of mixed ranking, as some would be of high and some of very low socio-economic status.

Urbanization and ties to agriculture

The degree of urbanization of the mother and the farming history of her family also were investigated on the theory that urbanization and distance from agricultural production would be proxy measures for distance from traditional culture. Table 6.6 indicates that more than half the mothers in all three locations had lived in towns or cities as children, yet close to half had been involved in farming and more than a third claimed that they planned to live permanently in the rural area in the future.

Table 6.6: Urbanization and ties to agriculture by location

Means (SD) and Percents

	Rural (N=20)	Semi-rural (N=74)	Urban (N=86)	Total (N=180)
Mother's present residence	11%	41%	48%	100%
Location of mother's residence as a child:				
Small village	35%	21%	7%	16%
Big village	5%	18%	18%	16%
Town	10%	21%	12%	15%
City	50%	41%	64%	53%
Mother's plan to live permanently in a rural area in future	50%	34%	31%	34%
Urbanization scale	2.0(.00)	3.6(.52)	5.3(.52)	4.2(1.22)
Child's mother				
Never farmed	25%	53%	55%	51%
Some farming	40%	36%	35%	36%
Mainly farming	35%	11%	9%	13%
Child's father				
Never farmed	10%	26%	54%	37%
Some farming	70%	57%	37%	49%
Mainly farming	20%	17%	9%	14%
Mother's father				
Never farmed	10%	13%	24%	18%
Some farming	30%	21%	34%	28%
Mainly farming	60%	66%	42%	54%
Mother's paternal grandfather				
Never farmed	0%	7%	12%	8%
Some farming	6%	16%	16%	15%
Mainly farming	94%	77%	72%	77%
Farming scale	6.2(1.8)	5.5(2.7)	5.5(2.9)	5.5(2.7)

More than half of the fathers in the present generation had engaged in some farming, though less than a fifth were mainly farmers, while more than half of the mothers' fathers and three-fourths of their grandfathers had been farmers. The farming history of the family members was summed to create a farming scale: which is the sum of the farming experience of the child's father and mother and the mother's father and her paternal grandfather. The mother's current and original locations were combined in a composite urbanization scale.

Mother's income, food expenditure, and wealth

Because of the length of the interview, income information was limited to food expenditure by source, and mothers' own earnings. Income information was collected by asking the mother to estimate in one of three exclusive ways (daily, weekly, or monthly) the following amounts: the mother's own net income; the father's contribution for food; the mother's contribution for food; and the total amount all others contributed for food. The interviewers had pocket calculators and helped mothers to make these estimations, particularly in converting all daily, weekly, and monthly amounts into single figures.

Per capita values were obtained by dividing by the number of persons of each age and sex eating from the family pot, converted into adult equivalent units. In polygamous families in which the father was present at least some of the time, the male adult equivalent unit representing his presence was divided by his number of wives.

After conducting logical checks and eliminating detracting outliers, the mother's own contribution to food expenditure was used to replace her reported income if her food expenditure was higher than her earnings. The mother's total budget was estimated as the sum of her earnings and the amounts she received for food expenses from the father and from others.

Table 6.7 shows the food expenditure and mother's income variables, illustrating the fact that the mother's own average earnings were highest in the rural group while the father's contribution to food expenditure was highest in the urban. Per capita food expenditure in the urban, however, was reported to be only 4 naira per week more than in the rural, a difference of 11 versus 15 naira. At the naira-to-US dollar exchange rate of about 8:1 prevailing at the time of the study, the families were spending on average US$1.60 per person per week on food.

Table 6.7: Sources and weekly amounts of household food expenditure by location

Means (SD), Percents and Ratios

	Rural (N=20)	Semi-rural (N=74)	Urban (N=86)	Total (N=180)
Father's weekly contribution to food expenditure				
0	26%	6%	5%	8%
1–10	26%	24%	15%	20%
11–20	27%	31%	18%	24%
21–30	11%	21%	20%	20%
31–40	5%	4%	23%	13%
≥41	5%	14%	19%	15%
Mean for those who contribute	16.9(10.7)	24.5(19.7)	32.7(26.1)	27.6(22.8)
Mother's weekly earnings	62.0(50.4)	31.7(31.3)	42.0(45.4)	39.9(41.5)
0	0%	3%	2%	2%
1–10	17%	16%	6%	11%
11–20	6%	22%	24%	21%
21–30	11%	27%	27%	25%
31–40	11%	11%	12%	12%
≥41	55%	21%	29%	29%
Ratio of mother's earnings:				
To father's contribution	17:1	3:1	8:1	7:1
To all other contributions	16:1	3:1	2:1	5:1
Mother's disposable income	77.0(55.3)	50.5(42.5)	64.5(48.6)	60.0(47.4)
1–10	6%	4%	6%	5%
11–20	11%	12%	5%	9%
21–30	0%	27%	4%	14%
31–40	6%	12%	16%	13%
41–50	0%	12%	13%	12%
51–60	28%	9%	9%	11%
61–70	17%	3%	15%	10%
≥71	32%	21%	32%	26%
Mother's disposable income per capita	21.3(17.3)	9.7(10.6)	12.2(14.7)	12.2(13.8)
0	0%	3%	2%	2%
1–5	17%	38%	31%	32%
6–10	17%	35%	38%	34%
11–15	11%	14%	10%	12%
16–20	22%	3%	5%	6%
≥21	33%	7%	14%	14%

	Rural (N=20)	Semi-rural (N=74)	Urban (N=86)	Total (N=180)
Mother's weekly contribution to food expenditure	18.3(23.6)	16.3(15.8)	26.1(33.4)	20.8(26.0)
0	0%	3%	2%	2%
1–5	32%	21%	18%	21%
6–10	21%	34%	22%	27%
11–15	21%	11%	12%	13%
16–20	0%	6%	4%	5%
21–25	16%	6%	18%	12%
≥26	10%	19%	24%	20%
Others' contributions to food expenditure	1.6(5.7)	0.2(1.0)	1.9(7.7)	1.2(5.6)
0	85%	95%	87%	90%
1–10	10%	5%	8%	7%
≥11	5%	0%	5%	3%
Total food expenditure from all sources	30.9(22.6)	38.0(24.7)	53.3(42.6)	44.1(34.9)
1–10	10%	5%	5%	6%
11–20	35%	26%	14%	21%
21–30	25%	22%	9%	16%
31–40	10%	15%	16%	15%
41–50	0%	11%	17%	12%
≥51	20%	21%	39%	30%
Per capita food expenditure	11.4(8.1)	11.0(7.0)	14.9(10.3)	12.8(8.9)
1–5	25%	32%	16%	24%
5–10	45%	30%	29%	30%
11–15	10%	14%	18%	16%
16–20	5%	14%	18%	15%
≥21	15%	10%	19%	15%

Socio-economic variables, child growth and development

Statistically significant socio-economic contrasts between the high and low developmental groups are reported in table 6.8. Most prominent in this table are the differences in mother's per capita income and the ratio of her earnings to the father's contribution to food expenditure.

The farming scale is significant whether or not the rural sample is included in the test. Yet farming experience of individual family members failed to reach significance. Most evidently lacking are the educational variables, of which the only marginally significant variable is the mother's ability to read Yoruba. One reason for the absence of educational associations is the tendency for more educated mothers to have higher per capita earnings (r=.2-.3; p<.01) and to work away from home (p=.081).

Mothers of the well-nourished children were more likely to have grown up in towns rather than big villages or cities and were less likely to live now in the rural location. They were significantly less likely to be living in a face-to-face dwelling and significantly more likely to have a monogamous husband. Yet they had on average more persons per room and a larger household, with more persons eating from the family pot. Differences in child status with respect to electrification and housing structure appeared secondary to rural-urban location, and consequently did not warrant further exploration.

Table 6.8: Selected socio-demographic and economic differences between developmental groups*

Means (SD), Percents and Ratios

	Low (N=69)	High (N=69)
Mother's education (years)	4.8	4.6***
Father's education (years)	7.0	6.8***
Mother reads Yoruba	50%	65%**
Mother grew up in a town (not big village or city)	6%	25%
Current residence:		
Rural	17%	1%
Semi-rural	46%	44%
Urban	36%	55%
Urbanization scale	3.8(1.2)	4.5(1.0)
Type of house:		
Face-to-face	84%	68%
Compound	6%	11%
Detached	10%	21%
Household size	5.1	5.8
Persons per room	0.30	0.26
Polygamous unions	55%	33%
Child's father never farmed	30%	43%
Farming scale	6.1	5.0
Father's weekly contribution to food expenditure (naira)**	25.0	28.2
Mother's weekly earnings	48.4	33.1
Ratio of mother's earnings to father's contribution	12:1	3:1

	Low (N=69)	High (N=69)
Ratio of mother's earnings to all other contributions	7:1	3:1
Mother's per capita earnings	14.89	9.1
Percent of mother's earnings spent on food**	53%	63%
Per capita food expenditure weekly (naira)**	13.2	13.4
Father's per capita contribution (naira)	7.4	7.8**

Note: * All contrasts significant at p<.05 except where indicated
          ** p<1
          *** Not significant

Logistic regression analysis

Table 6.9 presents three logistic regressions which represent the ability of the socio-economic subset of the data to predict the developmental category of the children. This table gives odds ratios with 95% confidence intervals and significance levels predicting the child's membership in the low developmental group. It shows the percentage of children correctly classified by each equation (concordant cells) and the overall significance level of the model (chi-square for co-variates).

No major differences in significant variables emerged from similar runs which included or excluded either the small rural sample or the purposive malnourished sample. To illustrate this fact, the second and third equations present the same model with and without the malnourished sample.

The natural logarithms of the economic variables are used in multivariate analysis, after adding 1 to prevent problems with 0 values. Out of hesitancy regarding the candour of income reporting, we checked the quality of all of the income and expenditure variables using robust regression (Minitab, REGRESS) to explore the associations between these variables, nutritional status, and MDI scores. This procedure produced almost exactly the same coefficients and significance levels as ordinary least squares regression.

The farming scale variable is the sum of the farming experience of the child's father and mother, the mother's father and her paternal grandfather, where 0 means never; 1, sometimes; and 2, always or mainly farmed. This near-normally distributed scale has a Chronbach's ALPHA for reliability of data, ranges from 0-12, has a mean of 5.5 and a SD of 2.7.

Dummy variables represent rural and urban location. The urbanization variable, with values from 1-3, combines location of mother's residence as a child with her current residence into an index of rural-urban mobility. All mothers currently living in the rural area, and those who have moved from urban childhoods to current semi-rural residence have values of 1. Mothers who grew up in big villages or towns and moved to Lagos city have values of 3. All others, including those who were born and remained in the city were assigned values of 2. These values reflect hypothesis building based on associations between the location variables and the growth status and test score variables. Children with values of 3 had the best and those with values of 1, the worst outcomes in exploratory analysis.

The first regression shows that higher per capita earnings of the mother and greater family farming experience increase the likelihood of a negative outcome in the child, whereas a monogamous father and an actively urbanizing family decreases this probability. Higher contribution to food expenditure by the father is positive but not statistically significant. The second and third models show that in the absence of the income variables, the mother's years of schooling enters negatively.

The odds ratios are the increase or decrease in probability of a negative outcome *per unit increase* in each independent variable. Thus, for mother's education in the second equation, an additional year of schooling increases the odds by 1.12. Cumulatively, this implies that six additional years of schooling approximately double the probability of a low outcome. Correspondingly, the probability of a child's falling into the low developmental group increases as the mother's per capita earnings increase and a rural child is somewhere between 7 and 14 times more likely to be in the low developmental group.

Table 6.9: Socio-economic predictors of low developmental group

	Odds	Ratio	Confidence Interval	Sig
Model I				
Intercept	1.05		.0–11.56	.97
Monogamous father	.37		.15–.92	.03
Farming scale	1.24		1.06–1.46	.01
Urbanization scale	.34		.16–.73	.00
Father's contribution per capita	.92		.55–1.55	.75
Mother's earnings per capita	1.88		1.01–3.50	0.4
Chi-square for covariates		29.9		

	Odds	Ratio	Confidence Interval	Sig
Model II with malnourished sample				
Intercept	.31		.10–.97	.04
Monogamous father	.26		.11–.63	.00
Farming scale	1.28		1.10–1.48	.00
Rural location	7.78		.83–72.92	.07
Urban location	.61		.27–1.37	.22
Mother's education	1.12		1.00–1.26	.04
Chi-square for covariates		31.6		
Model III without malnourished sample				
Intercept	.15		.04–.55	.00
Monogamous father	.25		.09–.71	.01
Farming scale	1.31		1.10–1.55	.00
Rural location	13.97		1.42–137.73	.02
Urban location	.63		.24–1.66	.34
Mother's education	1.15		1.00–1.31	.04
Chi-square for covariates		33.2		

Discussion

The presence of consistent significant relationships in this study is of relatively greater importance than their size as measured by the logistic procedure, given that the samples are not designed for determining population parameters and that not all relationships are linear. For example, the very strong negative relationship between mother's per capita earnings and the child's developmental status depends on the presence of mothers earning less than 12 and more than 50 naira per capita per week. When these mothers are excluded, a marginally significant positive correlation (p=.1) exists between WAZ of the child and his mother's per capita earnings.

The analyses in this section more strongly support the cultural distance hypotheses than the primary hypotheses of the study, as described in Chapter 1. Improvement in child status is most strongly associated with moves away from traditional agriculture as an occupation and from an earning pattern in which the mother and her children are the primary economic unit. These moves are toward a pattern in which the father lives more intimately together with and takes greater financial responsibility for his wife and children. We should not generalize from an analysis based on two-year-olds that mothers' intensive involvement in income generation is detrimental to her children. Mothers with high earnings may have children who are at greatest risk at the child-care intensive ages up to two or three years but who later benefit from greater maternal investment in schooling as well as nutritional advantages of more available food.

Chapter 7

Household structure and reproductive characteristics

Household structure is of importance to the psychological and material support that the mother receives and to her reproductive history, health and psychological state, all of which influence the growth and development of children ((Zeitlin *et al.* 1990, 43-52, 63-66, 72-78). It is for this reason that this study investigated this variable.

Family composition

Table 7.1 enters in detail into marital status and number of children by location. Three-fourths of the mothers classified themselves as married according to native law and custom and another 13% claimed to be cohabiting without being married. Very few were officially married (6%), divorced (2%) or single (2%). The interviewers in their debriefing session stated that only a more educated or enlightened mother would consider herself single, and then only if it was by her own choice that she did not live with the child's father. Whether or not he was married to another woman, if it was by his choice that he did not live with her she would consider herself married. In three-fourths of homes the father lived with the mother all the time. Two wives was the mode (79%) among the small rural group, while more than half (52%) of the semi-rural and two-thirds of the urban group were monogamous.

Given the significance of family structure to children's developmental outcomes, it is unfortunate that questions specifically concerning co-wives were omitted as sensitive information not considered necessary to the study. Polygamous husbands were less likely to live with their wives all the time (67% vs. 77%) and more likely to live with them less than half the time (20% vs. 7%). As expected, polygamous rural families tended to live together, with 81% of rural polygamous husbands always with their wives, compared to 61% of the semi-rural and 69% of the urban.

Table 7.1: Marital status and number of children by location

Percents

	Rural (N=20)	Semi-rural (N=74)	Urban (N=86)	Total (N=180)
Marital status:				
Single	0%	3%	2%	2%
Cohabiting	10%	22%	7%	13%
Married under the Marriage Act	5%	8%	5%	6%
Married by native law	80%	62%	85%	75%
Widowed	0%	1%	1%	1%
Divorced	5%	4%	0%	2%
Father lives with mother:				
All the time	79%	67%	80%	74%
More than half the time	0%	7%	4%	5%
Less than half the time	5%	16%	8%	11%
Rarely or never	16%	10%	8%	10%
Father's number of wives:	2.1(0.8)	1.7(0.9)	1.5(0.8)	1.6(0.9)
One	11%	52%	67%	55%
Two	79%	34%	19%	32%
Three	5%	10%	12%	10%
Four or more	5%	4%	2%	3%
Mother's number of children	3.2(1.6)	3.1(1.7)	3.4(1.7)	3.3(1.7)
One	11%	24%	12%	17%
Two	21%	14%	20%	18%
Three to five	63%	49%	56%	54%
Six or more	5%	13%	13%	12%
Father's number of children	6.2(8.7)	4.5(3.4)	4.5(3.4)	4.7(4.4)
One	10%	18%	11%	14%
Two	10%	11%	14%	12%
Three to five	50%	39%	48%	44%
Six or more	30%	32%	27%	30%
Fathers with more children than mother	42%	46%	33%	39%
Mother with more children than father	5%	6%	6%	6%

Only 22% of polygamous versus 16% of monogamous households claimed to have more than one adult woman member; and only 11% of polygamous versus 7% of monogamous women claimed to regularly share cooking duties. This suggests that only about 6% of polygamous women counted a co-wife as a member of the household. More detailed analysis suggested that living with a co-wife was more common in the semi-rural sample, in which 27% of polygamous versus 13% monogamous families had more than one adult woman, and less common in the urban sample, where 22% of polygamous versus 19% of monogamous families reported two adult women.

Table 7.2: Age composition of household by location

Means (SD) and Percents

	Rural (N=20)	Semi-rural (N=74)	Urban (N=86)	Total (N=180)
Men ≥ 18 years	0.9(0.5)	0.9(0.5)	1.1(0.7)	1.0(0.6)
None	17%	18%	11%	11%
One	78%	75%	75%	75%
Two or more	6%	7%	14%	14%
Women ≤ 18 years	1.1(0.3)	1.2(0.5)	1.2(0.5)	1.2(0.5)
None	15%	3%	1%	3%
One	70%	73%	79%	75%
Two or more	15%	25%	20%	22%
Boys 11–17 years	0.2(0.4)	0.3(0.6)	0.3(0.6)	0.3(0.6)
None	80%	74%	74%	75%
One	20%	21%	21%	21%
Two or more	0%	6%	5%	5%
Girls 11–17 years	0.3(0.4)	0.4(0.6)	0.4(0.7)	0.4(0.6)
None	75%	70%	66%	68%
One	25%	25%	25%	25%
Two or more	0%	5%	9%	7%
Children 6–10 years	0.6(0.6)	1.3(1.0)	1.0(1.0)	1.1(1.0)
None	49%	27%	35%	33%
One	47%	27%	39%	35%
Two	5%	38%	20%	26%
Three or more	0%	7%	6%	6%
Children ≤ 5 years	1.7(0.8)	1.6(0.8)	1.6(0.6)	1.6(0.7)
One	50%	54%	46%	49%
Two	40%	30%	51%	41%
Three or more	10%	16%	4%	10%
People eating from the same pot	4.6(1.3)	5.7(2.2)	5.6(2.2)	5.5(2.2)
Two	5%	3%	2%	3%
Three	15%	12%	12%	12%
Four to six	75%	54%	62%	60%
Seven or more	5%	32%	24%	25%

The number of wives varied by religious affiliation. Rates of monogamy were 68% for foreign Protestants, 59% for indigenous Protestants, 49% for Muslims, and 17% for the six rural Catholic families. By contrast 21% of foreign Protestant, 10% of indigenous Protestant, and 16% of Muslim families had three or more wives.

A third of the urban mothers and 42-46% of the semi-rural and rural reported that the child's father had more children than they had themselves, indicating children by other wives or liaisons. In only 6% of cases, the number of children of the mother was greater than that of the father. It is probable that not only these women but a significant percentage of other women had children from earlier liaisons.

Age composition of the households is presented in Table 7.2, showing that the average household had 1.8 children between the ages of 6 and 17 and 1.6 younger than five. Only 21% of the index children were first-born, and 17% were only children of their mothers. Yet in almost half of the families (49%) the index child was the only child younger than five years.

Mother's reproductive history and desired family size

Table 7.3 details by location the mother's height, weight, and body mass index (BMI). Rural mothers are on average shorter (p=.02) than semi-rural or urban. The urban when compared to the semi-rural and rural samples have the same proportions of thin mothers below BMI 19.8 (about 90% of weight-for-height) but have a significantly greater proportion of heavy women with BMI greater than 22.5 (41% versus 25%, p=.02).

According to Table 7.4, mean age at first birth (estimated by subtracting the age of the mother's oldest child from her reported age) was close to 20 years. Failure to account for mortality of first-born children increased this estimate by a small but unknown amount. This finding is not inconsistent with the Ondo State figure for median age of about 20 at first birth (DHS 1986).

Muslim mothers were on average two years younger than Christians at time of interview, although age at first birth was only 0.8 years younger for Muslims than Christians. Polygamous mothers were on average three years older than monogamous, reflecting the time needed to acquire a second wife and also the younger ages of the more educated mothers, who were more likely to have monogamous partners.

Table 7.4: Mother's reproductive history by location

Means (SD) and Per cents

	Rural (N=20)	Semi-rural (N=74)	Urban (N=86)	Total (N=180)
Mother's weight (kg)	50.6(7.6)	55.3(9.8)	56.5(10.5)	55.4(10.0)
<40	5%	0%	1%	1%
40–45	5%	10%	9%	9%
45–55	70%	45%	40%	45%
55–65	10%	30%	29%	27%
65–75	10%	11%	16%	13%
>75	0%	4%	5%	4%
Mother's height (cm)	156.7(5.2)	159.8(5.5)	159.5(5.0)	159.3(5.2)
<145	5%	0%	0%	1%
145–155	30%	19%	18%	20%
155–165	60%	67%	67%	66%
165–175	5%	13%	15%	13%
>175	0%	1%	0%	1%
Mother's BMI	21.5(5.2)	21.6(3.6)	22.2(4.0)	21.9(4.0)
<16	5%	1%	1%	2%
16–19	20%	18%	21%	20%
19–22	50%	43%	33%	39%
22–25	10%	23%	26%	23%
25–28	10%	10%	13%	11%
>28	5%	5%	7%	6%

Mean years of schooling of monogamous mothers was 4.9 versus 3.6 for the polygamous (p=.033). Similarly, monogamous fathers averaged 7.3 school years versus 5.9 for polygamous (p=.011). Yet age at first birth did not differ between polygamous and monogamous mothers. Age at first birth was relatively lower for mothers with 3-5 and 7-8 years of schooling (17.9 years) than for those with 0-2, 6, and 9-10 years (19.4), whereas the 16 mothers with 11+ years of school averaged 23.4 at first birth (p=.00001). The lower ages at first birth for the groups with incomplete primary and middle school education suggest that education was terminated by childbirth for some of these mothers. The findings with respect to age at first birth by religion, and for mothers with secondary education, closely resemble median figures reported for Ondo State (DHS 1986)

Table 7.5: Parental education, duration of breastfeeding and average birth interval by presence of sibling younger than index child

Means

	Child has younger sibling	Mother pregnant	No sibling, mother not pregnant	Total
Mother's education (years)	5.90	5.81	4.01	4.35
Father's education (years)	8.00	9.47	6.29	6.74
Duration of breast feeding (months)	11.70	12.40	15.30	14.70
Average birth interval (years)	1.7	2.21	3.03	2.84

Average duration of breast-feeding declined significantly with increasing urbanization (p=.0003) from 16.9 to 13.5 months. Both birth interval and length of breast-feeding decreased with increasing education of the mother and father. Table 7.5 present some of these associations.

Regression analysis indicates, however, that it is the father's education, increased financial dependence of the mother on the father and reduced months of breast-feeding that drive the decrease in birth interval, although mother's education is significant when father's education is not in the model. By contrast, mother's education and urbanization drive the reduction in breast-feeding. Higher per capita earnings of the mother also are associated with shorter breast-feeding.

A measure of ideal number of children was obtained from the number of children the mothers had already and the number more that they wanted, asked separately for boys and girls. The interviewers' probe for this question consisted of asking the mothers, "What do you tell God in your prayers?" Table 7.6 gives the number of additional children desired and ideal number, which was on average 5.8 (SD 1.8). Only 5% of the sample mothers had more than six children.

The total picture which emerged was thus:

The more children a woman had borne, the less educated she was, the higher her income, the younger she was (only marginally significant), the greater her number of co-wives, and the higher her ideal number of children, as shown in regressions in Table 7.7. Ideal number of children was 5.6 for wives of monogamous versus 6.4 for those of polygamous partners (p=.03). The data suggests that competition involving number of children among co-wives in polygamous settings pushed up their ideal for number of children.

Table 7.6: Additional children and ideal number of children by location

Means (SD) and Percents

	Rural (N=20)	Semi-rural (N=74)	Urban (N=86)	Total (N=180)
Girls desired	1.9(1.7)	1.3(1.1)	1.2(1.0)	1.3(1.1)
None	25%	30%	32%	30%
One	15%	25%	30%	26%
Two	35%	37%	29%	33%
Three or more	25%	8%	9%	11%
Boys desired	2.1(1.5)	1.6(1.2)	1.2(1.2)	1.4(1.3)
None	16%	25%	36%	30%
One	21%	18%	31%	25%
Two	32%	34%	21%	27%
Three or more	31%	23%	12%	18%
Total additional children desired	3.9(3.1)	2.9(1.9)	2.3(1.9)	2.7(2.1)
None	15%	17%	23%	20%
One	5%	9%	9%	9%
Two	15%	4%	25%	19%
Three	20%	16%	16%	17%
Four	15%	25%	13%	18%
Five	0%	12%	6%	7%
Six or more	30%	7%	8%	10%
Ideal number of children	7.0(2.6)	5.6(1.6)	5.7(1.6)	5.8(1.8)
One	0%	0%	0%	0%
Two	0%	4%	0%	2%
Three	10%	4%	3%	4%
Four	5%	13%	22%	17%
Five	10%	23%	20%	20%
Six	20%	28%	29%	28%
Seven	15%	16%	9%	13%
Eight or more	40%	12%	17%	16%

Use of family planning is illustrated in Table 7.8. Overall, about 13% of mothers claimed to use a family planning method currently and 28% to ever have used a modern method, with highest rates in the urban sample and for the pill. Specific methods used are listed in Table 7.9.

Logistic regression, shown in Table 7.10, for current use and any use of modern contraception, shows the following variables to be most important in influencing the use of family planning: reduced duration of breast-feeding; whether the mother had heard that she could use family planning, resume sexual relations, and continue breast-feeding without harming the baby; the mother's education; larger number of the mother's children; and short birth interval. Father's education and mother's wages also were significant and positively correlated with family planning use, although these are not represented in Table 7.10.

Table 7.7: Determinants of ideal number of children

	Dependent variables Ideal number of children		
Independent variables	**Model I**	**Model II**	**Model III**
Father's number of wives			
B	.29	.22	.18
Beta	.16	.12	.10
Sig T	.05	.13	.23
Mother's education			
B		−.07	−.08
Beta		−.16	−.17
Sig T		.04	.05
Per capita wages earned by mother			
B		.02	.03
Beta		.16	.22
Sig T		.05	.01
Age of mother (continuous variables reconstructed from categories)			
B			−.07
Beta			−.22
Sig T			.08
Mother's number of children			
B			.28
Beta			.26
Sig T			.05
Constant	5.47	5.66	6.80
Sig C	.000	.000	.000
Sig F	.05	.01	.06
Adjusted R^2	.02	.07	.08
N	155	155	143

Discussion of reproductive characteristics

The associations reported above reflect a population in an uneasy transition, engaged in replacing postpartum abstinence with the use of modern contraception but not yet displaying a mastery of the mechanisms involved. The associations between family planning use and larger total number of children indicate that contraception was used to limit family size towards the end of childbearing.

The associations between reduced birth interval, father's education, mother's dependence on his income, reduced breast-feeding, and the use of family planning confirm qualitative information regarding the problems caused by the postpartum taboo in an urban setting and difficulties encountered in the attempt to replace it with family planning.

By traditional standards, "good girls" were supposed to resist advances by their husbands during lactation; and good husbands were not supposed to insist. Educated men would be more monogamous in orientation and would tend to know that the postpartum taboo could be avoided. Mothers who were more dependent on their husband's incomes would be more compliant in yielding to their wishes to resume sexual relations, as they would be at greater risk if the husband sought gratification elsewhere. Many educated mothers apparently were cutting short the usual duration of breast-feeding, resuming marital relations, and attempting to maintain traditional birth intervals by using family planning, but with limited success.

Table 7.8: Mother's contraceptive practices by location

Percents

	Rural (N=20)	Semi-rural (N=74)	Urban (N=86)	Total (N=180)
Modern contraception ever used	5%	23%	37%	28%
Currently using	0%	9%	20%	13%
Currently using modern method or abstinence	10%	26%	42%	32%
Mothers who desire more children				
currently using modern method	0%	33%	15%	20%
currently using abstinence	33%	25%	30%	29%
Use of contraception can substitute for abstinence during breast feeding				
Mothers who have heard	70%	75%	78%	76%
Mothers who believe	41%	43%	50%	46%

Table 7.9: Knowledge & use of family planning methods by location

Percents

	Rural (N=20)	Semi-rural (N=74)	Urban (N=86)	Total (N=180)
Any method used previously	5%	23%	37%	28%
Any method used now	0%	9%	20%	13%
Breast feeding:				
Doesn't know method	10%	3%	6%	7%
Knows but has not used	25%	27%	24%	25%
Used previously	20%	53%	62%	54%
Uses method now	30%	16%	8%	7%
Pills				
Doesn't know method	50%	18%	15%	20%
Knows but has not used	45%	69%	61%	63%
Used previously	5%	9%	12%	10%
Uses method now	0%	4%	12%	7%
IUD				
Doesn't know method	70%	50%	23%	40%
Knows but has not used	30%	45%	67%	54%
Used previously	0%	1%	5%	3%
Uses method now	0%	4%	5%	4%
Condom				
Doesn't know method	65%	50%	32%	43%
Knows but has not used	35%	47%	58%	51%
Used previously	0%	3%	6%	4%
Uses method now	0%	0%	5%	2%
Injection				
Doesn't know method	60%	27%	18%	26%
Knows but has not used	40%	70%	79%	71%
Used previously	0%	3%	4%	3%
Tubal ligation				
Doesn't know method	65%	32%	35%	37%
Knows but has not used	35%	65%	65%	62%
Uses method now	0%	3%	0%	1%
Rhythm				
Doesn't know method	65%	47%	35%	44%
Knows but has not used	25%	32%	47%	39%
Used previously	5%	15%	11%	12%
Uses method now	5%	5%	7%	6%
Abstinence				
Doesn't know method	40%	22%	18%	22%
Knows but has not used	25%	31%	37%	33%
Used previously	25%	28%	19%	24%
Uses method now	10%	19%	27%	22%

	Rural (N=20)	Semi-rural (N=74)	Urban (N=86)	Total (N=180)
Foaming suppository				
Doesn't know method	75%	59%	51%	57%
Knows but has not used	25%	40%	45%	40%
Used previously	0%	1%	2%	2%
Uses method now	0%	0%	2%	1%
Diaphragm				
Doesn't know method	80%	71%	72%	73%
Knows but has not used	20%	27%	28%	27%
Uses method now	0%	1%	0%	0.6%
Cream				
Doesn't know method	95%	77%	65%	73%
Knows but has not used	5%	23%	35%	27%
Herb				
Doesn't know method	53%	60%	48%	53%
Knows but has not used	47%	38%	51%	45%
Used previously	0%	3%	0%	1%
Uses method now	0%	0%	1%	0.5%

A significant number of individual focus group members, possibly as many as one in ten couples, however, reported that they now began contraception and resumed marital relations one to four months postpartum without weaning the baby from the breast. This trend is suggested in the fact that family planning use was predicted by the mother's positive response to the question whether she had heard that sexual relations would not harm the health of the breast-feeding infant so long as the couple used family planning. Prohibition of sexual relations throughout lactation is very common among the Yoruba. Such postpartum taboos on sexual relations, believed to be universal in Africa in the pre-colonial era (LeVine *et al.*, 1990), were reinforced by the belief that semen entering the body during sexual relations poisoned the mother's milk. The institution of female circumcision may have made it easier for the woman to endure two to three years of sexual abstinence while she breastfed each child, and even to share a single room with her children for most of her life.

In response to postpartum abstinence, many monogamous Lagos husbands were claimed to have temporary affairs which increased their risks of contracting sexually transmitted diseases. Focus groups disclosed three maternal responses to the postpartum taboo:

(a) A minority of women abandoned the postpartum taboo, practised family planning, resumed marital relations in the early months' postpartum, and continued breast-feeding. These mothers believed that the family planning method would protect their baby from falling sick when sexual relations were resumed. They reported that it was the father's decision to take this new course of action.

(b) A larger minority appeared to stop breast-feeding their babies quite early, privately but not publicly admitting that they had stopped in order to resume relations. Oni's finding (1987) that use of family planning was negatively correlated with breast-feeding duration may reflect the practices of this group.

(c) The majority still claimed to practise traditional abstinence. They fatalistically denied that early resumption of relations combined with family planning and continued breast-feeding could protect their babies and keep their husbands faithful. These women's attitude was that their men sought other women regardless of their own availability. Some stated the fear that they and the baby might be exposed to diseases from resuming intercourse because the man had been running around, even if the semen didn't poison their milk. They appear vulnerable to peer pressure to stop breast-feeding earlier.

Table 7.10: Determinants of use of contraception

	Odds Ratio	Confidence Interval	Sig
Duration of breast feed	1.18	1.07–1.30	.00
Mother has heard use of contraception can substitute for abstinence during breastfeeding	5.89	.71–48.8	.09
Additional number of children desired	1.52	1.15–2.02	.00
Chi-square for covariates	28.0		

Co-wives compete for entitlement in polygamous families by bearing more children, as reflected in the relationship between ideal family size and number of the mother's co-wives. The fact that ideal family size increased with maternal income but decreased with greater maternal education suggests that children still were perceived by their mothers as an investment good, i.e. if one had more resources it would be both desirable and ultimately profitable for the future to invest in bearing more children; but that more educated mothers had a better understanding of the costs needed to prepare children for successful futures.

Family composition and child's nutritional and developmental status

As expected, all of the maternal anthropometry variables were significantly correlated with child anthropometry, except that height of the mother did not predict WHZ of her child. By contrast, the mother's height was her only physical measurement that was marginally significant with the child's Bayley score. Children scoring in the top tertile of the Bayley had mothers who were on average 1 cm taller than those in the bottom tertile, while children in the tallest HAZ tertile had mothers averaging 3 cm taller than those in the shortest tertile.

Child deaths experienced by the mother showed a relationship to child growth and development opposite to that usually found in non-African populations (Table 7.11). ANCOVA was carried out comparing the child's HAZ, WAZ, and MDI for mothers with none versus any child deaths, with mother's age and her height, weight and education as covariates (respectively in the three analyses). The analysis showed that mothers who had experienced child deaths had children who were significantly taller (.4 SD in HAZ, after adjusting for co-variates), marginally heavier, but not scoring higher on the Bayley tests than those whose mothers had never experienced a child death.

Decreased birth interval was negatively correlated with HAZ (p=.035). Table 7.11 shows the child's HAZ as determined by the mother's height, body mass index, and birth interval from the index child to the next child (p=.049).

Short birth intervals introduce new family stresses

Short birth intervals were found in this study to be relatively common, and were perceived as a problem by low-income focus group members, placing a strain not only on child care but on all parental resources. Some Lagos women working in the modern sector, however, expressed a preference to have their children densely spaced and then to be free of childbearing. This attitude suggests a shift towards interest in family limitation, a departure from the older ideology of unlimited good in childbearing.

Table 7.12 shows the family composition and reproductive variables which differ between the high and low developmental groups. The high group were significantly more likely to have the father living with the family, and to have one wife as noted earlier. Significantly fewer well-developing two-year-olds had pregnant mothers. The mothers of those index children who already had younger siblings were found to have higher BMIs, which could have protected the growth and development of their more closely spaced children. A traditional birth succession with two children below five and two between 6 and 11 was significantly more common among high than low developers. Significantly more high-group families also had two adult women living in the house and a total family size of six to nine members.

Table 7.11: Influence of birth interval on child's height

Percents

Independent variables	Dependent Variable HAZ
Mother's body mass index	
B	.03
Beta	.10
Sig T	.14
Mother's height	
B	.05
Beta	.25
Sig T	.0003
Birth interval (years)	
B	.23
Beta	.13
Sig T	.05
Constant	−12.11
Sig C	.0000
Sig F	.0003
Adjusted R^2	.08
N	199

The structure and composition of the traditional family was determined by the age composition and living arrangements of members. When the postpartum taboo guaranteed that all children were spaced about three years apart with inevitable gaps caused by infant and child mortality, together with extended family members, the ratio of adults to children and of older to younger was relatively dependable.

With respect to nutritional status alone, there was a tendency for children of mothers wanting four or fewer children and for those wanting exactly six children to be better off than mothers desiring either five, or seven or more. This tendency reached statistical significance for WAZ. This is a curious result in need of greater investigation.

Developmental status relationships

Increased rates of stunting have been found to be associated with shorter birth intervals in other studies. Linear growth retardation would be caused by maternal depletion due to short pregnancy intervals, a combination of reduced breast-feeding and higher morbidity rates, and reduced resources and quality of attention available to the child.

However, the presence of a younger sibling did not appear to reduce the mother's proximity for the Nigerian study children. Children with younger siblings were just as likely as those without to stay with their mother when she worked at home, although they were marginally less likely to accompany her to the worksite.

The negative relationship between short birth interval and linear growth is a second major reason for the lack of positive associations between parental education and more promising child outcomes, since increasing education has tended to decrease birth intervals through concomitant reductions in postpartum abstinence and in breast-feeding.

These negative relationships also counterbalance potentially positive associations between contraception and nutritional status, since the parents most likely to contraception were those with reduced birth intervals and reduced breast-feeding.

Families as units of change

Families with five to seven members, with two adult women, and with children at each rung of the traditional birth ladder have better child outcomes than families of smaller and larger sizes. Those with longer birth intervals also have better outcomes. These facts suggest that there may be value in looking at the family as a whole rather than at individuals as units of change, and as the unit of analysis for positive deviance. The findings with respect to child spacing also tend to confirm Harkness and Super's (1989) developmental niche hypothesis.

**Table 7.12: Family composition and reproductive differences
between developmental groups***

	Low (N=69)	High (N=69)
Father lives with family		
All the time	64	70
More than half the time	2	6
Less than half the time	13	9
Rarely or never	20	6
Number of wives		
One	42	67
Two	40	20
Three or more	17	13
Birth interval below index child		
Younger sibling	12	10
Mother pregnant	14	3
No sibling, not pregnant	74	87
Household composition		
Two children under 5	33	54
Two 6–11 year olds	12	26
Two adult women	9	23
Number of family members		
Less than or equal to four	71	29
Five to seven	31	69
Eight or more	55	45
Mother's physiological indicators**		
Weight	54.6(10.7)	56.7(8.7)**
Height	150.3(5.7)	160.5(4.7)**
Body Mass Index	21.8(3.9)	22.0(3.3)***

* Significant at p<.05
** Significant at p<.1
*** Not significant

It is likely that family structures are closely attuned to the social conditions of production, considered in the broadest sense to include not only working conditions *per se* but the manner in which units of residence configured as families compete to take advantage of production opportunities. These conditions, and cultural ideologies that support them, provide scripts for family life with regard to child care and training. The greater adaptiveness of monogamy with urbanization is an example of a change in family structure that is strongly supported by a new cultural ideology.

As will be seen further in Chapter 8, changes in family structure which precede changes in the cultural script and ideology appear to have negative effects on child care. These changes alter the cast of traditional players in the care and enculturation of the child without corresponding adaptive changes in the scripts governing family and community life. Structural distance, without corresponding cultural distance, from traditional lifestyles tends to breed dysfunction, in a manner analogous to an attempt to introduce a new computer system without providing a new manual.

Interventions with a focus on family would by definition consider these aspects. Definitions of family health that included family structure could potentially define dysfunctional families as units requiring treatment with the same urgency that infectious illness is treated in the individual. Parents also might find such an approach more motivating than individual short-term interventions, as they already think of their children in the context of the family's future well-being, rather than of their children primarily as individuals.

In addition to monogamy, already included in the socio-economic status cluster, this section contributes only one significant variable–presence of the father living with the family - to the logistic regression models predicting membership in the high or low developmental groups. In effect, the paradoxical links between parental education and income, and reduced breast-feeding, birth interval, and time for maternal care, cancel out potential benefits of the variables commonly considered to measure the demographic transition. The father's presence is included in the next round of logistic analyses in Chapter 8.

Child care arrangements

Differences in care by location

The types of child care assistance and the physical circumstances of child care available to the mother are preconditions for the quality of care she is able to provide. Alternate child care arrangements were investigated in terms of the child's physical proximity to the mother, the location of the care, and the persons who regularly served as alternate caretakers. Table 8.1 displays the variables measuring the mother's physical accessibility to her child by location. Sixty-four per cent of mothers worked at least part of the time at a distance from the home, while about a fourth worked at home and 12% were at a shop or stall near but separated from the house.

More than half of the two-year-olds usually accompanied their mothers to work. Only 31% of children still were carried on the back for one or more hours daily. Most no longer were "backed" or were carried for less than one hour, only to calm them briefly, to put them to sleep, or occasionally to transport them. Urban children were less likely to be backed (23%) compared to the semi-rural and rural (32-35%).

More than half the mothers (62%) took either no days or one day off per week. They claimed to leave their two-year-olds for an average of 3.2 hours per day while they worked. When mothers worked around the house, 39% of the two-year-olds usually stayed in their sight, while 24% usually went away. This behaviour was not affected by whether there was a younger sibling of the index child or a new pregnancy.

Shifts with urbanization included the following tendencies: for the mother to take fewer days off from work; for the child to accompany the mother to the worksite, as more urban mothers worked away from home; for reduced carrying of the child on the back; and for the child to stay near the mother when she worked at home.

Differences in work and care locations by developmental group

Table 8.2 presents differences in mothers' physical accessibility to the child by developmental group. Children in the high group were significantly more likely to have mothers who worked either at home or near the home with no day or one day off, and were significantly less likely to usually leave their mothers' sight when she worked at home.

Table 8.1: Mother's physical accessibility to child by location

Means (SD) and Per cents

	Rural (N=20)	Semi-rural (N=74)	Urban (N=86)	Total (N=180)
Proximity of mother's workplace:				
At home	32%	23%	24%	24%
Shop/stall near but separate from home	5%	6%	19%	12%
Away from home	16%	44%	45%	41%
Away from and at home	42%	27%	12%	22%
Away from and near home	5%	0%	0%	1%
Child usually goes to work with mother	44%	50%	62%	55%
Two-year-old is carried on back:				
Never or occasionally	65%	69%	77%	72%
≥ 1 hour daily	35%	32%	23%	28%
No. of days mother takes off work per week:				
None	0%	19%	23%	19%
One	47%	38%	47%	43%
Two	24%	27%	25%	26%
Three	29%	16%	5%	12%
Child is left with someone else while mother works (hours)	3.8(5.8)	3.8(5.0)	2.7(2.9)	3.2(4.3)
0	25%	24%	26%	25%
1–2	45%	42%	43%	43%
3–5	15%	10%	16%	14%
6–8	0%	10%	7%	8%
9–11	10%	10%	0%	5%
Where child stays when mother works at home				
Usually with her	30%	31%	48%	39%
Sometimes with her	35%	43%	33%	37%
Usually goes away	35%	26%	19%	24%

Children who accompanied their mothers to the worksite at a distance from the house were less well nourished than those left at home. Mental development, and overall development, however, appeared to be closely linked to the degree to which the mother kept her child in her company when she was able. Of children with mothers working at a distance from home, 35% of those who accompanied the mothers to work still were backed, compared to 21% of those who remained at home.

Mothers working at home or close to home took fewer days off than those working at a distance; and those taking fewer days off had lower earnings than those who took off more days. Therefore, fewer days off appeared to indicate a lower rather than a higher work commitment.

Table 8.2 Mother's physical accessibility to child by developmental group*

	Low (N=69)	High (N=69)
Where mother works:*		
Home	21	30
Near home	9	15
Away or both away and at home	70	55
Where child stays when mother works at home**		
Usually in sight	32	42
Sometimes stays in sight	40	42
Usually goes away	28	16
Two-year-old is carried on back:		
No or only occasionally	64	81
Yes $\geq$ 1 hour daily	36	19
Number of days mother takes off work per week:		
0–1	57	72 (p=.065)
2–7	43	28

* Differences reach statistical significance when home and near home are contrasted with any time away

** Differences reach statistical significance when usually and sometimes with mother are contrasted with usually away.

Two-year-olds still carried on the back for one or more hours daily were significantly worse off on WAZ and MDI. The most significant differences, however, were in PDI, with average values of 100 versus 105 for regularly backed and no-longer or only occasionally backed children (Table 8.3).

Analyses investigating the combinations of the mother's working location and the child's location while she worked are presented in Table 8.4, which show the children's nutritional and developmental status outcomes for 12 care conditions. Group means for each of the care conditions were divided as nearly as possible into quartiles (see Appendix A for mean values and group assignment). The number from 1 to 4 in each cell represents the quartile ranking of the group mean.

The mother's work location was: away from home, at a stall or shop nearby, or at home. When not working at home, the mother could either leave the child behind, or take him with her. At times when the mother was working at home, the child could be within her view rarely, sometimes, or usually.

This table displays both developmental and nutritional indicators in order to illustrate that certain conditions relatively favourable to nutrition are less favourable to mental development and vice versa. In addition to WHZ, WAZ, HAZ, ZPOSDEV1, MDI and PDI, the mother's per capita earnings (ranked according to group mean values of the logarithmic transformation), and her years of education are included.

A 4++ notation is given to a group of seven children whose mental development scores averaged above 100, therefore increasing their developmental composite scores as well.

Children usually in sight of their mothers when the mothers worked at home showed a tendency to do better than those who did not, particularly with respect to the positive deviance score and to mental development. As noted above, whether or not the child stayed in sight did not depend on the presence of a younger sibling or the pregnancy status of the mother.

The worst-off group of children overall were the 29 whose high-earning mothers worked away from home and took the children to the worksite, but did not usually keep them in their company when working at home. An almost opposite high- ranking group were the 27 whose moderately high-earning and well educated mothers worked away and left the children behind, but when they were home kept in close contact with the children.

Next best were 40 children with low-earning mothers* working at home, in families where the child usually or sometimes stayed near the mother while she worked. The 15 in similar circumstances who did not stay near their mothers did not fare so well.

Contradictory effects are visible in the relatively high nutritional status but low MDIs of 17 children who stayed home but did not stay with their mother when she was home, compared to the very poor nutrition but relatively good cognitive test scores of 13 who went to work with their mothers and also stayed with her when she worked at home.

Table 8.3: Daily back-carrying of two-year-olds and child outcomes

	Means (SD) and percents		
	Not or only occasionally backed	Backed ≥ one hour daily	Sig
Weight-for-age Z Score	−1.70(.99)	−1.96(1.05)	.07
Height-for-age Z Score	−2.25(1.14)	−2.40(1.10)	.48
MDI	93(11.7)	90(10.4)	.03
PDI	105(15.4)	100(15.1)	.01
Mother working away from home			.07
Child accompanying mother	65%	35%	
Child remaining at home	79%	21%	

Primary and secondary caretakers

Mothers were read a comprehensive list of caretakers and asked whether each of them usually, sometimes, or rarely cared for the child while the mother worked or was away. The usual supplementary or alternate caretaker was considered primary. Persons described by the mother as sometimes taking care of the child were considered secondary caretakers.

The primary caretakers were ranked in the analysis through a process of hypothesis testing, and by the developmental status of their charges. Hypothesis testing was carried out for inductive and descriptive purposes. The hypotheses, drawn from the focus groups and the ethnographic study, were that care by siblings or a housemaid in the traditional 9- to 12-year-old child caretaker age group and by close adult female relatives would be best, while care by unrelated female friends of the mother would be worst. Cut-off points — for example, the choice of 9 (rather than 7 or 8) years as the lower limit for desirable sibling care — were derived from the data. Primary and secondary caregivers were ranked according to the developmental status of their charges if the ranking matched the prior hypotheses.

Where more than one primary caretaker was named, the child was considered to have the one with the highest ranking according to this previous procedure. It was assumed that the highest-ranking primary caregiver would set the standard for the quality of care the child received from other primary caregivers, and would fill in for the others. Primary caregivers of about equal rank were then grouped together if they provided care in socially similar circumstances. Thus mothers and 3-8 year old siblings are grouped together. Table 8.5 shows the primary and secondary care categories, as ranked, by location.

Children with adult male primary caretakers did particularly well. While not hypothesized, this finding was not a surprise considering the role of adult males in food allocation noted earlier in Section 4.6.1, and the better* outcomes found in monogamous homes in which fathers provided relatively more support. In fact, adult male caregivers were not more frequent in monogamous than in polygamous homes. Adult males usually were not the only primary alternate caretaker listed for the child.

Table 8.5: Child's caretakers in addition to mother ranked according to child outcomes by location

Means (SD) and Percents

	Rural (N=20)	Semi-rural (N=74)	Urban (N=86)	Total (N=180)
Primary alternative caretaker:				
Adult male	5%	12%	18%	14%
9–12 year old sibling or housemaid	10%	15%	16%	15%
Other female relatives	15%	14%	8%	12%
Grandmother	35%	31%	18%	26%
13–21 year old sibling	5%	5%	10%	7%
Mother alone or 3–8 year old sibling	25%	12%	14%	14%
Female friend of mother	5%	11%	17%	13%
Secondary alternate caretaker:				
3–8 or 9–12 year old sibling	30	24	13	19
Adult male	5	15	18	15
13–21 year old sibling	15	4	6	6
No secondary care	15	27	31	27
Female friend or relative	35	32	33	32
Number of alternate caretakers:				
Many primary, no secondary	0%	4%	6%	5%
Two primary, no secondary	15%	37%	38%	35%
Many primary, many secondary	10%	4%	4%	5%
One primary, no secondary	15%	16%	21%	18%
No primary, one secondary	55%	31%	25%	31%
No primary, no secondary	5%	8%	5%	6%
Quality of child care scale	.60(1.5)	.30(1.7)	.28(1.9)	.19(1.8)

The grandmother was sole primary caretaker and joint primary caretaker with another family member in addition to the mother with about equal frequency. Child outcomes were better when the grandmother was not the sole primary caretaker. Children in the primary care of 13- to 21-year-old siblings did relatively poorly on all measures. The number of such siblings (possibly half-siblings) was greater in polygamous households.

Secondary caretakers were ranked according to the mean developmental level of the children in their care, using ANCOVA to control for the rank of the primary caregiver. Outcomes were good when 3- to 12-year-old siblings served as secondary caretakers.

Table 8.6: Child's caretakers in addition to mother ranked according to child's outcomes by developmental group

Means (SD) and percents

	Low (N=69)	High (N=69)
Primary alternative caretaker:		
Adult male	6%	22%
9–12 year old sibling or housemaid	9%	19%
Other female relatives	13%	14%
Grandmother	27%	20%
13–21 year old sibling	10%	6%
Mother alone or 3–8 year old sibling	19%	10%
Female friend of mother	16%	9%
Secondary alternate caretaker:		
3–8 or 9–12 year old sibling	17%	29%
Adult male	13%	17%
13–21 year old sibling	6%	6%
No secondary care	28%	22%
Female friend or relative	18%	13%
Number of alternate caretakers:		
Many primary, no secondary	0%	9%
Two primary, no secondary	25%	46%
Many primary, many secondary	3%	4%
One primary, no secondary	20%	10%
No primary, one secondary	41%	26%
No primary, no secondary	12%	4%
Quality of child care scale	.78(1.5)	.86(1.8)

In addition, the total number of primary and secondary caregivers also was ranked through hypothesis testing. Hypotheses were that too little care (no primary caretaker aside from the mother) or too fragmented and less committed care (many secondary caretakers) would be bad, and that more primary caretakers would be good. Outcomes were best for those children with two or more primary and no secondary caretakers, and as might be expected were worst for those with no supplemental caretakers at all.

Apparent trends with urbanization were greater participation in both primary and secondary care by adult males; greater reliance for primary care on female friends and 13-21 year-old siblings, and less on grandmothers or other adult female relatives; and less secondary care overall.

A composite child care quality variable was created by applying a Z-score transformation to the primary care, secondary care, and number of caretakers variables in table 8.5 and to the composite ranking in the far right hand column of Table 8.4. These Z-scores were then summed, giving full weight to primary caretakers and number of caretakers, and half weight to secondary caretakers and the care condition ranking from Table 8.4. Values for this variable are shown by location in Table 8.5.

Differences in primary and secondary caretakers by developmental group

Table 8.6 shows the relative frequency of the ranked primary and secondary caretakers and number of caregivers by developmental group. Most striking for primary care is that 15% of the low group versus 41% of the high had an adult male or 9-12 year old sibling or maid as primary caretaker, while 45% of the low versus 25% of the high had the mother alone, very young siblings, teenaged siblings, or female friends.

With regard to number of caretakers, 25% of the low versus 55% of the high group had two or more primary caretakers, while 53% of the low versus 30% of the high had no primary caretaker.

Logistic regression analysis

Table 8.7 shows the results of logistic regressions in which the child care quality variable was added to the socio-economic variables presented earlier in Table 6.9, while removing the father's contribution to food expenditure which was not significant. The other variables remain significant with about the same odds ratios, while the number of children correctly classified increases by about 8% and the chi-square for covariates almost doubles.

Model II adds child care quality to the second model in Table 6.9, along with the log of the number of hours for which the mother leaves the child when she goes to work and a 0/1 categorical variable indicating whether the father lives with the family more or less than half the time. These additions increase the per cent of children correctly classified by 11%.

Table 8.7: Socio-economic and child care quality predictors of low developmental group

	Odds ratio	Confidential interval	Sig
Model I:			
Intercept	.26	.02–3.26	.29
Monogamous father	.29	.11–.80	.01
Farming scale	1.28	1.08–1.52	.00
Urbanization scale	.46	.21–1.02	.05
Mother's earnings per capita	2.59	1.24–5.41	.01
Quality of child care scale	.52	.38–.71	.00
Chi-square for covariates		56.7	
Model II			
Intercept	5.08	.32–81.09	.24
Monogamous father	.15	.04–.55	.00
Farming scale	1.30	1.07–1.57	.01
Quality of care scale	.51	.35–.73	.00
Rural location	12.45	.69–225.27	.08
Urban location	.54	.17–1.65	.27
Mother's education	1.21	1.02–1.44	.03
Father lives with family less than half the time	.27	.08–.91	.03
Hours mother is away from child at work	.35	.12–1.03	.05
Chi-square for covariates		49.7	

An important finding from this model is that entry of the quality of child care variable does not detract from but rather increases the significance of the other independent variables. The fact that the number of hours the mother habitually leaves the child is associated with better outcomes suggests that mothers carry the two-year-old along to work as a last resort.

Discussion

Child care was not monetized in a scheduled manner in this population, though food, services and other contributions were exchanged and monitored over the long term.

Every woman in the rural traditional community would have her turn to contribute to and to benefit from communal child care. The commonly occurring child housemaids or houseboys traditionally did not receive wages but were taken care of, fed, educated to some degree, and taught skills and manners. When there was a money transfer, it might be saved by the employer to be given as a lump sum at the end of the service. While older housemaids now have salaries in addition to room and board, they still tend not to have fixed working hours.

With urbanization, adult female relatives became less available as caretakers. Female friends lack the same level of commitment to the child, and cannot count on reciprocal care for their children, given that families living in low- income urban housing frequently change neighbourhoods. This is a situation in which the assumption that adequate child care is a free good is no longer valid. The cast of characters has changed but new scripts, which monetize child care and limit childbearing, are only gradually emerging.

One adaptive response to reduced community child care in the urban area appears to be keeping the young child closer to the mother. Whether an individual two-year-old actually stayed close probably depended on the family's living space, the mother-child attachment, the mother's strategy of investing in children, and her levels of stress and fatigue.

The findings that very young children were worse off nutritionally if they travelled with the mother to a worksite at a distance from the home reinforce the conclusion that alternate care is desirable for such children, even when their mothers labour in the informal rather than the formal sector. Of policy concern in these findings is the fact that care which increases the child's separation from the mother without providing adequate stimulation may be likely to improve nutrition at the expense of mental stimulation.

The findings that two-year-olds who still were carried regularly on the back fared worse than those who had come down from the back, and that mothers who took their children to work were more likely to back them, reflect a complicated situation. Lighter, less mature children would be more likely not yet to have graduated from the back. On the other hand, mothers who took their children far from home would need to back them there, and this need could have contributed to the child's malnutrition in earlier months, when the cultural ideal of avoiding a heavy child, (see *wuwo* in Chapter 4) could have led to food withholding.

If only nutritional factors were at play, growth differences should be most apparent. The fact that Bayley scores differed more than nutritional indicators between the backed and non-backed has more serious implications. This finding implies that backed children, who are passively immobilized, do not receive the motor stimulation and perhaps verbal that they need between 1-2 years of age. Earlier findings had shown extreme motor delays in always-backed children of vendors, with a mean walking age of 19 months compared to 10 months for children of a non-backed elite group.

Prolonged backing, which may foster the precocity of the young infant and facilitate exclusive breast-feeding in the early months, becomes as age-inappropriate for the older infant as would be continued exclusive reliance on breast-feeding. The educational message from the findings with regard to backing is simple: Do not regularly back your child for long periods after a certain age. However, determining that critical age will require further research.

Chapter 9

Health, sanitation and hygiene

The health and health treatment covariables were collected to serve as control variables for the central analyses. As this survey was not a morbidity study, precise epidemiological methods were not followed. While the data in this section reflect the children's levels of illness, they do not qualify as morbidity surveillance data with the exception of the past-two-week prevalence of symptoms of illness.

Child's illnesses by location

Mothers were asked about their child's illness history in two simple ways. First they were read a list of serious conditions and symptoms and asked whether the child had the condition now, or had ever had it in the past. The question used the Yoruba term "*nisin*", which means now-a-days or recently, but is translated as "now" in the tables. Thus the reported current rates of serious conditions reflect the caretaker's perceptions of an unspecified time window extending back from the immediate present. In the second question, the mothers were asked if the child had had symptoms of runny nose, cough, diarrhoea or fever at any time during the past two weeks.

Table 9.1 presents, by location, the caretaker's report of both the child's history of severe illness during his lifetime to date, and the child's illnesses however minor in the preceding two weeks. Highest illness rates were reported for malaria and fever, and for severe diarrhoea or dysentery. Only 20% of children were claimed never to have had malaria and 44% never to have had severe diarrhoea. Thirty-five per cent of the children had had measles; 7-8% kwashiorkor or marasmus (to their mother's knowledge); and 14% convulsions, usually accompanying fever (possibly in the presence of calcium deficiency). Only 31% were reported to have been completely healthy during the previous two weeks.

Table 9.1: History of child's illness by location

Means (SD) and Percents				
	Rural (N=20)	Semi-rural (N=74)	Urban (N=86)	Total (N=180)
Whooping cough				
Still has it now*	20%	3%	1%	4%
Had it in the past	10%	5%	11%	8%
Never had it	70%	92%	88%	88%
Pneumonia				
Still has it now*	25%	0%	0%	3%
Had it in the past	5%	3%	2%	3%
Never had it	70%	97%	98%	94%
Severe malaria				
Still has it now*	5%	8%	2%	5%
Had it in the past	85%	80%	69%	75%
Never had it	10%	12%	29%	20%
Other illnesses				
Still has it now*	10%	0%	0%	1%
Had it in the past	40%	49%	47%	47%
Never had it	50%	51%	54%	52%
Diarrhoea or dysentary				
Still has it now*	10%	7%	7%	7%
Had it in the past	60%	51%	44%	49%
Never had it	30%	42%	49%	44%
Frequent passing of worms				
Still has it now*	15%	0%	1%	2%
Had it in the past	15%	12%	14%	13%
Never had it	70%	88%	85%	85%
Measles				
Still has it now*	20%	0%	0%	2%
Had it in the past	45%	38%	27%	33%
Never had it	35%	62%	73%	65%
Kwashiorkor (leg swellings)				
Still has it now*	25%	0%	0%	3%
Had it in the past	10%	3%	6%	5%
Never had it	65%	97%	94%	92%
Marasmus (being very thin)				
Still has it now*	20%	0%	0%	2%
Had it in the past	10%	5%	2%	5%
Never had it	70%	95%	98%	93%

	Rural (N=20)	Semi-rural (N=74)	Urban (N=86)	Total (N=180)
Convulsions				
Still has it now*	10%	1%	0%	2%
Had it in the past	30%	12%	7%	12%
Never had it	60%	87%	93%	86%
Severe skin or other infections				
Still has it now*	20%	10%	7%	9%
Had it in the past	65%	61%	45%	54%
Never had it	15%	30%	48%	37%
Number of different illnesses the child has suffered from:	5.5(3.3)	3.5(1.6)	2.9(1.6)	3.4(2.0)
0 – 2	6%	13%	30%	20%
3 – 4	33%	53%	53%	50%
>4	51%	34%	17%	30%
Child's health status in past two weeks				
Healthy	20%	22%	42%	31%
Runny nose or cough	25%	36%	33%	33%
Diarrhoea with or without cold	10%	12%	7%	9%
Fever (with or without symptoms)	45%	32%	19%	27%

* Yoruba *nisin*, equivalent to "now", "nowadays", "recently".

Sources of treatment

Table 9.2 shows variables regarding the mother's treatment of illness, and her child's well-baby visits and growth monitoring. The majority of mothers took their children outside the home for treatment of fever, and the facilities most accessible to them were modern health clinics and pharmacies. A scale for quality of treatment was constructed by awarding points for seeking outside treatment for fever and seeking this treatment from a health clinic or private doctor rather than any other treatment source, for example a medicine store or chemist.

The fact that 80% of mothers reported that their children have been weighed is evidence both of some growth monitoring activity and of receptiveness to growth monitoring, although only 17% had weight charts in the home.

Sanitation and hygiene

Table 9.3 displays observations regarding household sanitation and water source, the methods the mothers used for cleaning their children's feeding bottles, and the percentages observed to wash hands before eating and use a clean dish in the feeding observation. From these variables a sanitation and hygiene scale was created, including presence of faeces or a dirty floor and water source.

Table 9.2: Mother's treatment practices for child illness by location

Means (SD) and Percents

	Rural (N=20)	Semi-rural (N=74)	Urban (N=86)	Total (N=180)
Where child is taken for treatment of fever				
Treated at home	50%	30%	24%	29%
Taken for outside treatment	35%	46%	45%	44%
Treated at home and taken for outside treatment	15%	23%	31%	26%
Other	0%	1%	0%	1%
Types of treatment most accessible to home				
Babalawo	0%	5%	12%	8%
Herb sellers	32%	10%	8%	10%
Pharmacist	16%	55%	35%	44%
Private doctor	5%	1%	11%	7%
Health clinic or hospital	47%	28%	34%	31%
Types of treatment on which family most relies				
Babalawo	0%	11%	5%	7%
Herb sellers	32%	13%	11%	14%
Pharmacist	16%	17%	6%	12%
Private doctor	5%	5%	12%	8%
Health clinic or hospital	47%	54%	66%	59%
Number of times child taken for check-up when not ill				
0 – 7	90%	76%	73%	76%
≥ 8	10%	24%	27%	24%
Child was weighed at clinic	47%	75%	91%	80%
Child has weight chart				
No	63%	60%	41%	51%
Yes, at clinic	32%	28%	36%	32%
Yes, at home	5%	12%	23%	17%
Quality of treatment scale	1.2(0.9)	1.5(1.0)	1.7(0.9)	1.6(0.9)

Health and hygiene by developmental group

Half of the children in the low group were said to have suffered from diarrhoea or fever during the preceding two weeks (Table 9.4), compared to 28% of the high group. None of the high group had suffered from kwashiorkor, and only 3% from marasmus, while of the low, 19-20% had experienced one or both of these conditions.

Table 9.3: Sanitation and hygiene indicators by location

Means (SD) and Percents

	Rural (N=20)	Semi-rural (N=74)	Urban (N=86)	Total (N=180)
Debris on floor, inside or out				
Animal faeces	50	15	2	13
Human faeces	0	1	0	1
Spoiled food	5	7	6	6
Other	75	65	67	67
Any wet or muddy areas inside the compound	30	31	80	54
Any safety hazards inside the home	40	25	34	31
Source of water:				
Stream	74	1	1	9
Well	5	19	1	9
Rain or tank	0	13	1	6
Borehole	5	28	0	12
Tap	16	39	96	64
Cleaning of feeding bottle				
Washed with cold water	6	4	1	3
Washed with boiling water	0	6	1	3
Washed with soap and water	33	6	6	9
Washed with soap and water, put in boiling water	39	70	37	51
Soaked in cold water and Milton or strong salt solution	22	14	55	35
Observed feed				
Hands were washed	15	10	8	9
Clean dish was used	100	93	98	96
Sanitation and hygiene scale	2.9(1.0)	3.9(1.0)	4.1(0.7)	3.9(0.9)

Thirty-six per cent of mothers of children in the low group had taken their children to the clinic when not ill eight or more times, compared to 23% of those in the high group (Table 9.5). Possibly the greater clinic attendance reflects the increased anxiety of mothers whose children tended toward malnutrition and experienced more diarrhoea than the high group. However, the overall quality of treatment scale for the two groups was not significantly different.

Table 9.4: History of serious child illness by developmental group

Means (SD) and Percents	Low (N=69)	High (N=69)
Severe diarrhoea or dysentery		
Still has it now*	12	3
Had it in the past	52	45
Never had it	36	52
Frequent passing of worms		
Still has it now*	7	0
Had it in the past	9	13
Never had it	84	87
Kwashiorkor		
Still has it now*	12	0
Had it in the past	7	3
Never had it	81	97
Number of illnesses episodes in past two weeks	3.2(2.0)	2.1(1.2)
Child's health status in past two weeks		
Healthy	29	37
Runny nose or cold only	20	35
Diarrhoea or fever	51	28

* Yoruba *nisin*, equivalent to now, nowadays, recently

Poor home hygiene and use of untreated water did not preclude a child's being in the high group, although low group households scored lower overall on sanitation and hygiene (Table 9.6) Of interest in this table is the cleaning of the feeding bottle, with the simple and inexpensive technique of soaking in strong salt or mild chlorine solution twice as common in the high as in the low group.

Table 9.5: Mother's treatment practices for child illness by developmental group

Means (SD) and Percents

	Low (N=69)	High (N=69)
Where child is taken for treatment of fever		
Treated at home	32%	28%
Taken for outside treatment	41%	45%
Treated at home and taken for outside treatment	27%	26%
Other	0%	1%[p-71]
Types of treatment most accessible to home		
Babalawo	18%	3%
Herb sellers	13%	6%
Pharmacist	41%	51%
Private doctor	10%	9%
Health clinic or hospital	18%	31%
Types of treatment on which family most relies		
Babalawo	12%	6%
Herb sellers	16%	10%
Pharmacist	10%	14%
Private doctor	7%	9%
Health clinic or hospital	54%	61%[p-53]
Number of times child taken for check-up when not ill		
0 – 7	64%	77%
≥ 8	36%	23%
Quality of treatment scale	1.5*1.0)	1.6(0.9)

Logistic regression analysis

Table 9.7 adds the total child illnesses variable to the previous models. The quality of treatment variable is not included here, as although it was significant in predicting lower total morbidity, it did not reach statistical significance in predicting developmental outcomes.

Model I adds total morbidity to Model II of 8.7, thereby increasing the percentage of correctly classified children to 88% and the chi-square for covariates to 64%. Model II similarly improves upon the preceding Model II, after removing the log value of the hours the child is left while mother works. With recent or long-term illness represented, variables in the two models combine in Model III to correctly classify 90% of the children.

Table 9.6: Selected sanitation and hygiene indicators by developmental group

Means (SD) and Percents

	Low (N=69)	High (N=69)
Debris on floor, inside		
Animal faeces	18	5
Other	77	60
Source of household water		
Stream	19	2
Well, rain, tank or borehole	19	28
Tap	62	70
Cleaning of feeding bottle		
Soaked in cold water and Milton or strong salt solution	23	46
Sanitation and hygiene scale	3.7(0.9)	4.1(0.9)

Access to foods tended to be a communal right within traditional society, structured as a built-in system of increasing in-kind rewards for seniority within the system. These rewards operated as incentives to continue to serve and maintain the system. Traditional rewards to senior Yoruba management were analogous to better quality food and service and more prestige.

Table 9.7: Total illnesses added to predictors of low developmental group

	Odds ratio	Confidential interval	Sig
Model I:			
Intercept	.04	.00–.72	.03
Monogamous father	.32	.11–.92	.03
Farming scale	1.32	1.10–1.58	.00
Urbanization scale	.50	.23–1.10	.08
Mother's earnings per capita	3.22	1.46–7.11	.00
Quality of child care scale	.54	.40–.74	.00
Total child illnesses	1.60	1.10–2.32	.01
Chi-square for covariates	63.6		
Model II			
Intercept	.28	.01–7.26	.43
Monogamous father	.17	.05–.61	.01
Farming scale	1.41	1.14–1.74	.00
Rural location	.84	.25–2.85	.78

Urban location	18.52	.78–438.30	.07
Mother's education	1.29	1.06–1.56	.01
Father lives with family less than half the time	.24	.06–.89	.03
Quality of child care scale	.51	.35–.75	.00
Total child illnesses	1.51	.93–2.47	.09
Chi-square for covariates		58.9	
Model I:			
Intercept	.00	.00–.07	.00
Monogamous father	.32	.09–1.12	.07
Farming scale	1.47	1.17–1.86	.00
Rural location	.84	.23–3.12	.79
Urban location	13.47	.94–193.89	.85
Mother's earnings per capita	4.10	1.51–11.08	.00
Quality of child care scale	.50	.34–.75	.00
Total child illnesses	1.58	.99–2.52	.05
Chi-square for covariates		60.5	

Chapter 10

Feeding practices

Breast and bottle feeding

The study obtained simple diet histories and food frequencies for the children.

Diet history questions regarding infant feeding centred on breast and formula feeding, methods of weaning from the breast, and age of introducing the adult diet. Only one mother did not initiate breast-feeding and only two were no longer breast-feeding at three months. Yet, as shown in Table 10.1, 93% of mothers also used a feeding bottle, usually with a supplementary formula or milk mixture.

Focus group discussions indicated that the normative pattern was to introduce the bottle during the naming ceremony shortly after birth and to withdraw the bottle with the introduction of staple foods. Overall, almost ninety percent of women started the bottle before 1 month of age, about 52% specifying "at the naming ceremony" held at eight days, 13% "at birth," and 24% "before one month."

Almost all mothers had given water to their infants, with 89% stating that they had boiled it. However, almost one third of the rural women, 79% of whom used stream or well water, were not treating it before using it to prepare feeds for their babies. Urban women, almost all of whom had piped water, were far more likely to boil water used for the baby's feeds.

Breast-feeding was prolonged and terminated on average at 15 months overall, ranging from 17 in the rural to 14 in the urban sub-samples. Bottle feeding stopped at an average of 10 months.

Associations between breast-feeding and development

Table 10.2 illustrates the fact that no bivariate associations were visible between duration of breast or bottle feeding and developmental status. As will be shown later in Table 10.18, multivariate analysis shows this appearance to be misleading, because analysis methods which controlled for confounding variables revealed significant benefits of longer breast-feeding. Moreover, there was a significant difference (p=.017) in duration of breast-feeding between the bottom (14.2 months) and top (15.9 months) MDI tertiles.

Table 10.1: Infant feeding history of child by location

Means (SD) and Percentages

	Rural (N=20)	Semi-rural (N=74)	Urban (N=86)	Total (N=180)
Ever breastfed	100	100	100	100
Duration of breast feeding (months)	17.1(3.7)	16.1(3.8)	13.7(4.9)	15.1(4.3)
0-6	0%	2%	10%	5%
7-12	15%	27%	35%	29%
13-18	55%	56%	46%	52%
>19	25%	9%	7%	10%
Still breastfeeding	5%	6%	2%	4%
Ever bottle fed	85%	96%	95%	93%
Age stopped bottle feeding (months)				
<1	94%	93%	82%	88%
1	6%	4%	11%	7%
2-6	0%	3%	7%	5%
Age stopped bottle feeding (months)	9.6(6.7)	9.1(5.5)	10.8(5.7)	9.9(5.7)
0-6	30%	37%	24%	30%
7-12	40%	40%	45%	42%
13-18	0%	13%	19%	15%
>19	20%	7%	8%	9%
Still bottle feeding	10%	3%	3%	4%
Household treatment of water used in feeding infant				
No treatment	32%	10%	7%	11%
Boiled	68%	90%	93%	89%

Dissynchronous weaning practices were significantly more common in the low than in the high developmental group (51% vs 33%, p =.039); and twice as many low as high group infants (24% vs 12%) were reported to have stopped breast-feeding by themselves (p=.06).

The study found unexpected relationships between sudden weaning and nutritional status. The suddenly weaned group were significantly better off in WAZ and WHZ than the gradually weaned. Worst off were the 4% whose mothers had adopted neither strategy; and best off were the children of three highly educated mothers who reported gradually reducing breast-feeding and then stopping in one day.

Clinicians have often reported cases where the nutritional or health problems of a child brought for health treatment appeared to date from sudden, traumatic weaning from the breast. Such clinical findings could have led to an incorrect generalization that sudden weaning is worse for the child than gradual weaning, when on a population basis the suddenly weaned children may have had better nutritional status. Particularly in our sample, for whom nutrient dense foods were scarcely affordable and for whom the idea of withholding food dovetailed with concepts of moral training, gradual reduction of breast-feeding may have been a form of food deprivation not compensated for by giving the child increased amounts of other foods.

Another mechanism by which gradual weaning could have negative effects might occur if a power struggle developed between an undernourished child and her mother over access to the breast. Gradual withdrawal of the child's "breast privileges" could prolong a stressful interaction pattern. These paradoxical findings highlight the lack of clarity of definition of the term "gradual weaning," like most terms applied to breast-feeding (Armstrong 1991), and the need to conduct concept testing of the specific meaning of weaning advice given in health education messages.

Table 10.2: Infant feeding history by developmental

Means (SD) and Percentages		
	Low (N=69)	High (N=69)
Ever breastfed	100.0%	100.0%
Duration of breastfeeding (months)	15.1	14.4%
Age stopped breastfeeding (months) 0-6	7%	6%

	Low (N=69)	High (N=69)
7-12	32%	3%
13-18	44%	49%
>19	13%	10%
Still breastfeeding	4%	1%
Ever formula (bottle) fed	94%	96%
Age started bottle feeding (months)		
<1	88%	85%
1	9%	7%
2-6	3%	8%
Age stopped bottle feeding (months)	9.6%	10.3%
0-6	32%	27%
7-12	42%	48%
13-18	12%	16%
>19	11%	6%
Still bottle feeding	3%	3%

Dissynchronous weaning

A number of practices used in weaning the child from the breast were identified and these are shown by location in Table 10.3, divided into the subcategories gradual weaning and sudden weaning. We use the term dissynchronous to refer to practices which may be most likely to occur when there is a lack of mutuality between mother and child regarding the timing of weaning. Many of the practices are applied by mothers who are ready to stop breast-feeding, with children who resist leaving the breast.

Another form of dissynchrony may be indicated by the mother's statement that the child "stopped by himself," suggesting that the child's timing was ahead of the mother's expectation. This interpretation is supported by the fact that the average age of weaning of the 23 self-stoppers was 11 months, four months earlier than the sample mean. The mean age of under one year among these children, a period when true self-weaning is rare, suggests that mothers were readily taking some passing disturbance in the baby's breast-feeding behaviour, such as nipple confusion, teething, distractibility, or a sudden nursing strike, as the baby's desire to stop breast-feeding altogether.

Overall 39% of children were reported to have experienced dissynchronous weaning from the breast. A mistake in wording of a question regarding whether the mother had "put the baby to sleep" to break off the breast-feeding probably caused underreporting of the use of the antihistamine syrup phenergan or beer to make the child sleep. While some mothers did put the child to sleep for a day starting in the early afternoon (as was asked in the Yoruba questionnaire), more used a sleeping draught at bedtime for a few nights to keep the child from waking and crying for the breast. There was no difference in the rate of dissynchronous weaning practices between gradual and sudden weaning.

Table 10.3: Practices used in weaning child from breastfeeding by location

Means (SD) and Percentages				
	Rural (N=20)	Semi-rural (N=74)	Urban (N=86)	Total (N=180)
Dissynchronous weaning				
Put the child to sleep for the day	5%	7%	5%	6%
Send the child away from the house for a while	25%	18%	13%	17%
Have child sleep away from mother	10%	3%	4%	4%
Rub bitter substance on breast	20%	16%	6%	11%
Child stopped by self	25%	11%	12%	13%
Other	0%	10%	13%	10%
Percent with one or more form of Dissynchronous weaning	50%	42%	34%	39%
Sudden weaning of children who did not stop by themselves (stopped in one day, did not reduce breastfeeding before-hand (N=151)	40%	56%	72%	62%
Gradual weaning (reduce breastfeeding, did not stop in one day	40%	46%	28%	37%
Reduced breastfeeding and also stopped in one day	0%	6%	1%	3%
Had not reduced or stopped at time of study (N=6)	5%	4%	2%	3%

The term gradual weaning refers to reduction in number of daily breastfeeds over a period of time, phasing them out gradually. Gradual weaning is distinguished from sudden weaning, which means cutting out all breastfeeds in one day. Of the 151 mothers in the total study population who had terminated breast-feeding without the child stopping by himself, 34% reported that they reduced breast-feedings and did not stop in one day (gradual weaning), 60% did not reduce breast-feedings and weaned in a single day (sudden weaning), while three mothers had both reduced feedings beforehand and then weaned in a day. Six were still breast-feeding.

Age of introducing the adult diet

This survey did not investigate the introduction of the *ogi* (fermented dilute, white maize pap) given almost universally from about five months, or of the expensive multinational brand-name baby cereals, which appeared to be used by a few in token amounts or used as bottle admixtures.

There was reported imprecision by mothers in distinguishing between token introduction of tastes of the food and introduction of large quantities. Since infant feeding generally starts with tastes and gradually increases, this imprecision is to be expected. In the case of the very hot chilli peppered soups and stews which characterize Yoruba cuisine, however, the imprecision is greater. Focus groups and participant observation by the project team members drew attention to the Yoruba practice of accustoming babies to pepper by introducing a daily dab of soup from the mother's finger into the baby's mouth at three to five months, expecting the baby first to cry and after some days or weeks to learn to tolerate the sting.

Beans and peppered soup were first and meat was last to be introduced. Highly significant rural-to-urban differences in average age of introduction reached a maximum of almost five months for fish and egg (treated as a single category). Regression analysis (Table 10.4) entering rural and urban location as separate dummy variables with education revealed that both location and the mother's education were significant predictors.

Associations with nutritional status and developmental group

Table 10.5 reveals sharp differences in mean age of introducing foods by developmental group. Especially marked was the earlier introduction of protein foods to the children in the high developmental group, who received fish, eggs, and meat two to three months earlier than low scorers.

Table 10.6 displays Spearman's non-parametric correlation coefficients between the ages of introduction and the individual outcome measures, illustrating the fact that the associations are far stronger with the Mental Development Index than with the growth variables or the Physical Development Index.

Table 10.4: Determinants of age of introducing adult foods

Independent variables	Dependent variables Age of introducing adult foods
Rural location	
B	1.95
Beta	.14
Sig T	.04
Urban location	
B	-2.55
Beta	-.32
Sig T	.000
Last year of school completed by mother	
B	-.14
Beta	.13
Sig T	.05
Constant	13.49
Sig C	.000
Sig F	.000
Adjusted R2	.17
N	201

Timing of introduction of adult foods

The very large rural-to-urban shift towards earlier introduction of foods, as well as the universal adoption of bottle feeding, indicate that this population does not generally resist changes in infant feeding practices. Given such major shifts in certain dietary areas, where there is resistance to change this would tend to confirm the presence of deep-seated cultural values of the type surrounding meat (see Section 10.4 below). The shift to earlier introduction of family foods appears less likely to be a reflection of commercial marketing than does the widespread adoption of infant formula, although food introduction could be influenced by the marketing of commercial baby cereals.

Table 10.5: Ages in months when adult foods were introduced by developmental group

	Low	High	Sig
Carbohydrate rich foods such as *eba, amala*	12.6	11.6	.165
Soup with pepper	9.5	9.1	.593
Protein rich foods such as beans, fish, eggs			
Beans	13.0	10.3	.0002
Fish and Eggs	10.9	9.1	.028
Meat	12.7	9.2	.0001
	15.1	12.3	.003
Age at which fish and eggs were introduced (months)			
0-6	16	36	
7-11	21	22	
12-13	26	30	
14-24	37	12	
Age quartile at which fish and eggs were introduced (months)			
0-6	31	69	
7-11	48	52	
12-13	47	53	
14-24	76	24	

The finding that age of introduction of adult foods is much more strongly associated with the cognitive test score than with growth or physical development may imply that micronutrients in the protein-rich foods have protective value for cognitive development even if the quantities are not sufficient to maintain normal growth. Alternatively, it could be that the same mothers who introduce family foods early are much more likely to provide cognitive stimulation for their children.

Table 10.6: Ages of food introduction and child outcomes correlation coefficients

Spearman's r values, p values in parentheses

Food	Beans	Fish & egg	Meat	Mean for protein
HAZ	-.03(.356)	-.11(.064)	-.08(.139)	-.06(.176)
WAZ	-.07(.150)	-.15(.017)	-.07(.151)	-.11(.059)
WHZ	-.13(.034)	-.13(.037)	-.04(.290)	-.10(.369)
PDI	-.06(.203)	-.12(.051)	-.08(.433)	-.15(.581)
MDI	-.18(.005)	-.24(0001)	-22(.001)	-.25(.0001)
ZPOSDEV1	-.15(.019)	-.25(.0001)	-.15(.004)	-.23(.001)

Food frequencies

Mothers were read a pre-tested list of foods normally consumed in the Nigerian diet and asked whether the child ate each food: daily (five or more times per week); weekly (up to four or more times, almost every week); monthly (one to two times a month); occasionally; or never. The impatience of the mothers during the pre-test of more detailed frequency questions led to the adoption of this simplified format.

Responses were converted for analysis into estimated servings per week. It was suspected that frequencies were sometimes exaggerated by the mother for the sake of good appearance or because it was not customary to make such fine-grained time distinctions. A few mothers had responded to many food items with a hearty, "Every day! Yes. Every day!"

Tables 10.7 and 10.8 show the average frequency per week with which children consumed the individual food items and common food groups by location and overall. The total frequency averaged 91.1 servings per week, ranging from 87.7 for the semi-rural to 94.3 for the urban.

This difference was not statistically significant. Of the overall total, starchy staples made up 27.5 servings, including 7.3 for cassava products, 6.1 for rice, 6 for African yam products, and 4.6 for maize (excluding hard roasted corn on the cob). Foods of animal origin totalled 15.2 and legumes (including all kinds of beans and peanut products and melon seeds) 14.9; hence total protein foods totalled 30.1. Servings of green vegetables and stews containing them were reported 8.9 times per week; all fruits 9.2 times, of which 4.3 were oranges; and snacks, 7.1 times.

In general, there was a tendency for home grown farm products, products of on-farm manufacture, and products with high mark-ups in urban versus rural markets, such as pawpaw (papaya), guava, yam, palm oil, and *egusi* to be eaten more frequently by the rural group, whereas street foods, such as steamed bean cake (*moin-moin*), plantain, and biscuits, and northern ethnic foods, beef kebabs (*suya*) and soft Nigerian cheese (*wara*) to be more common in the diets of the urban children.

In aggregate, the urban diet tended towards significantly more frequent consumption of protein foods, both from legume and animal sources, more snacks, less of cassava and maize staples, and higher ratios of protein foods, both to carbohydrates and to total servings.

Table 10.7: Number of servings of common foods per week by location

Food (N=180)	Means			Sig	Total
	Rural (N=20)	Semi-rural (N=74)	Urban (N=86)		
Rice	6.5	6.0	6.2	0.47	6.1
Cold maize pap	2.3	2.0	1.2	0.09	1.6
Hot maize pap	3.0	2.5	2.6	0.92	2.6
Maize Porridge	1.1	0.3	0.1	0.0003	0.3
Maize on cob	1.6	0.8	0.7	0.64	0.9
Yam	4.5	2.7	3.8	0.004	3.4
Pounded Yam	0.5	0.7	0.5	0.24	0.6
Yam flour gel (amala)	0.9	1.0	3.0	0	2.0
Cassava meal gel (eba)	5.3	4.7	2.9	0	3.9
Cassava floor gel (lafun)	0.3	1.7	1.7	0.0003	1.5
Cassava meal (garri)	3.0	2.2	1.3	0.006	1.9
Plantain	0.6	1.2	2.2	0	1.6
Okra	1.7	2.1	1.9	0.51	1.9
Greens (efo)	2.4	1.9	2.0	0.64	2.0
Greens, slippery leaf (ewedu)	2.7	3.0	3.0	0.47	3.0
Greens with melon seeds	2.6	1.9	1.8	0.67	1.9
Melon seeds (egusi)	2.7	1.7	1.2	0.02	1.6
Seeds of fruit (apon)	0.8	0.4	0.8	0.12	0.6
Meat soup	3.1	4.2	4.2	0.02	4.3
Pepper soup	0.6	0.2	0.4	0.02	0.4
Bitter leaf soup (obeekero)	0.6	0.2	0.1	0.004	0.4
Groundnut soup (gbegiri)	0.5	0.1	0.9	0.0005	0.2
Palm oil	0.9	0.1	0.3	0.002	0.3
Beans	3.7	3.7	3.8	0.9	3.8
Fried bean cake (akara)	1.7	1.9	2.0	0.73	1.9
Steamed bean cake (moin-moin)	1.3	1.8	2.5	0.009	2.1
Manu	0.02	0.5	0.5	0.11	0.4
Groundnuts	1.5	1.6	3.0	0.0005	2.2
Fried groundnut meat	2.0	1.9	2.6	0.18	2.3
Groundnut snack	1.3	1.7	2.1	0.94	1.9
Meat	0.9	1.5	0.8	0.2	1.1
Chicken	0.2	0.4	0.3	0.27	0.3
Fish	4.7	5.5	5.0	0.4	5.2
Snails	0.2	0.4	0.2	0.36	0.3
Pieces of meat (suya)	0.05	0.1	0.8	0	0.4
Soft cheese (wara)	0.02	0.1	0.3	0.04	0.2
Milk	1.4	2.3	3.1	0.002	2.6
Eggs	2.4	2.0	2.5	0.08	2.3
Animal hide	1.3	1.6	1.5	0.72	1.5
Intestines	0.7	1.1	1.2	0.19	1.1
Oranges	3.8	4.2	4.6	0.33	4.3
Pawpaw	2.1	1.5	0.8	0.03	1.2

Food (N=180)	Rural (N=20)	Semi-rural (N=74)	Urban (N=86)	Sig	Total
Banana	1.1	1.3	1.9	0.05	1.6
Pineapple	1.5	0.5	0.8	0.05	0.8
Other fruit	2.5	1.6	0.9	0.7	1.5
Biscuits	1.1	2.2	3.5	0	2.7
Sweets	1.3	2.6	1.7	0.02	2
Commercial drinks	.2	2.5	2.2	0.54	2.3
Other snack foods	0	0.3	2.9	0.19	1.5

Because of potential respondent bias with regard to meat, two totals of animal food intake were constructed, one with and one without meat.

Differences in weekly frequency of consumption by top and bottom per capita food expenditure quartile and by developmental group are presented in table 10.9. Totals ranged from 88.6 servings per week for the lowest versus 93.3 for the highest food expenditure quartiles, and were almost identical for the low and high developmental groups (89.0 servings versus 90.9). Both significant and non-significant differences are retained in these tables for their descriptive interest, and significance levels are given.

Foods eaten significantly more often in the top food expenditure quartile included *suya*, milk, pineapple, biscuits, sweets, and plantain, and total foods of animal origin (all $p < .05$), and eggs, pawpaw, *amala*, and meat soup ($p > .05$ and $< .16$). Those eaten more often by the lowest quartile were *robo* (a snack made from the cake from which peanut oil had been pressed), *egbo* (maize porridge), hot and cold maize pap, total maize-based staples, *gari* (cassava meal usually drunk diluted with water), total cassava products and palm oil ($p < .16$). Except for *robo*, these "poor" foods were more commonly eaten in the rural area where food expenditure was lower.

The high developmental group more frequently consumed milk, oranges, bananas, plantain and biscuits ($p < .05$) and *suya*, tripe, chicken, sum of animal foods (excluding meat), beans and "other" snacks ($p > .05$ and $< .1$). The low group had more maize porridge, hot pap, maize-based staples, and vegetable and *egusi* ($p < .1$). The high group reported significantly higher ratios of protein foods to carbohydrates ($p = .05$) and of animal foods excluding meat to total servings ($p = .03$). As in the case of age of food introduction, differences tended to be slightly more significant between top and bottom MDI tertiles than between WAZ or HAZ tertiles.

Table 10.8: Number and ratios of servings per week of selected categories of food by location

Means and ratios

Food (N=180)	Rural (N=20)	Semi-rural (N=74)	Urban (N=86)	Sig	Total
Maize as staple	6.4	4.8	3.9	0.05	4.6
Cassava products	8.5	8.6	6.0	0.0001	7.3
Green vegetables	9.4	8.9	8.7	0.88	8.9
Accompaniments	18.5	15.9	17.5	0.24	17.0
Legumes	11.7	13.4	16.9	0.006	14.9
Animal foods including meat	12.1	15.1	16.1	0.04	15.2
Animal foods excluding meat	11.2	13.6	15.3	0.007	14.1
Protein foods including meat	23.9	28.5	32.9	0.007	30.1
Protein foods excluding meat	22.9	27.0	32.2	0.0022	29.0
Fruits	11.7	9.0	8.8	0.44	9.2
Snacks	4.4	7.3	7.5	0.05	7.1
Total servings*	89.7	87.7	94.3	0.2	91.1
Total carbohydrate foods*	31.0	26.7	27.3	0.38	27.5
Radio of protein to carbohydrate foods	0.83	1.1	1.2	0.002	1.13
Ratio of protein to total servings	0.26	0.3	0.34	0.003	0.31
Ratio of animal foods including meat to total servings	0.13	0.17	0.07	0.07	0.17
Ratio of animal foods excluding meat to total servings	0.12	0.15	0.16	0.03	0.15

Children diagnosed as malnourished

Mothers were asked in the section on serious illness whether their children had experienced marasmus or kwashiorkor, and a total of 29 (14%) were reported either previously or currently to suffer from one of these conditions.

The overall quality of these children's diets was lower, as illustrated in Table 10.11. These children were likely to be of lower birth order, with younger mothers in polygamous marriages, and to have been born after shorter birth intervals.

Table 10.9: Number and ratios of servings per week of selected categories of food by location by food expenditure quartile and developmental group

Means and ratios

Group Food	Food expenditure quartile			Developmental		
	Low	High	Sig	Low	High	Sig
Maize as staple	5.2	3.8	0.01	5.1	3.7	0.06
Cassava products	7.7	7.2	0.16	8.1	7.3	0.24
Green vegetables	8.9	8.4		9.2	8.7	0.67
Accompaniments	16.9	17.0	0.86	17.7	16.5	0.91
Legumes	14.7	14.3	0.73	15.0	15.6	0.64
Animal foods including meat	13.7	17.3	0.01	14.2	15.7	0.35
Animal foods excluding meat	12.5	16.4	0.01	12.8	14.8	0.09
Protein foods including meat	28.4	31.0	0.32	29.3	31.2	0.5
Protein foods excluding meat	27.2	30.7	0.28	27.9	30.4	0.29
Fruits	9.2	9.5		7.4	8.7	0.05
Snacks	5.7	8.1	0.11	6.0	7.4	0.07
Total servings	88.6	93.3	0.65	89.0	90.9	0.58
Total carbohydrate foods	28.1	27.0	0.25	28.3	26.7	0.5
Ratio of protein to carbohydrate foods	1.0	1.2	0.07	1.0	1.2	0.05
Ratio of protein to total servings	0.3	0.32	0.15	0.3	0.33	0.12
Ratio of animal foods including meat to total servings	0.15	0.19	0.003	0.16	0.17	0.27
Ratio of animal foods excluding meat to total servings	0.14	0.17	0.002	0.14	0.16	0.03

Discussion of food frequencies

The differences between the high and low developmental groups in frequency of consumption of the various foods tend to confirm long-standing observations that protein-rich foods are critical to child development in Southern Nigeria. Several findings are particularly worth noting.

Total legumes did not differentiate between the high and low groups overall, but did distinguish between those who had and had not been diagnosed as malnourished. This suggests that the bean foods, while not promoting rapid growth, protect against overt protein=calorie malnutrition. Protein-rich animal foods may protect against malnutrition through the micronutrients they contain rather than through the protein per se (Golden 1989).

The fact that the animal food total and protein-to- carbohydrate ratio had slightly higher associations with the MDI than with the growth variables reinforces the idea introduced previously that micronutrients in the protein-rich foods may have protective value for cognitive development even if the quantities are not sufficient to maintain normal growth. To the extent that this is true, poor parents should be encouraged to give whatever small amounts they can afford of these foods to their children, even if a growth impact would not be detectable from these quantities. Lower threshold levels are not known for the various types of child development. Just as 10 mg of Vitamin C can ward off scurvy, although far more than this amount is beneficial, it may be that token amounts of high-quality foods can protect functional capacity.

The possibility that the oil and vegetables in the stews in which the animal foods are served and the staples eaten with them make more difference than the animal foods themselves is not likely, given that the total servings of soups and stews did not differ significantly between developmental groups.

Because of the very low protein content of cassava, discussed in Chapter 5, greater consumption of cassava was hypothesized to be linked to poorer developmental outcomes. In fact the poorer outcomes were linked to the maize staples *ogi, eko*, and *egbo*, which are very low in caloric density. Cassava although low in protein is the highest of the staples in calories per volume eaten.

Given the increasing reliance on cassava products for food security in Nigeria, it was reassuring not to find unfavourable associations with cassava. Alternatively, the degree of reliance upon cassava could have been underreported by the mothers who considered it to be a low status feed. Meat, fish and eggs were however regarded as very high status foods in general.

Meat distribution and moral training

Several items on the nutrition questionnaire investigated the mothers' attitudes and practices with respect to meat distribution within the family, especially to two-year-old children.

While fish was more commonly eaten than meat, the ethnographic study revealed that slivers of fish given to the children could be even smaller than pieces of meat, because cooked fish can be divided easily. Meat was selected because it was the food most frequently and emotionally referred to when parents articulated the traditional value system with regard to children, food, and spoiling.

Table 10.10: Dietary and socioeconomic characteristics of children reported to have experienced kwashiorkor or marasmus

	Children with K/M (N==28)	Children without (N=182)	Sig
Mean selected servings of selected foods			
Cold maize pap	2.3	1.5	.10
Hot maize pap	3.6	2.5	.10
Yam	2.5	3.4	.03
Plantain	1.1	1.6	.10
Vegetable and egusi	2.5	1.9	.05
Akara	1.5	2.0	.09
Moin-moin	1.7	2.1	.04
Groundnuts	1.6	2.3	.03
Kuli-kuli	.8	2.0	.04
Suya	.4	.5	.07
Milk	1.9	2.6	.04
Intestines	.6	1.1	.06
Biscuits	1.8	2.6	.03
Sweets	1.1	2.2	.06
Mean weekly total servings of selected food categories			
Maize as staple	6.2	4.3	.04
Legumes	12.3	15.2	.03
Animal foods including meat	13.1	15.0	.11
Animal foods excluding meat	12.2	13.9	.12
Protein foods including meat	25.4	30.2	.03
Protein foods excluding meat	24.5	29.1	.03
Snacks	4.7	7.2	.02
Ratios			
Protein to carbohydrate foods	.87	1.14	.004
Protein foods to total servings	.27	.32	.004
Animals foods including meat to total servings	.07	.15	.17
Animals food excluding meat to total servings	.10	.13	.15
Meat portion for two-year old from family share	.08	.07	.21
Socioeconomic characteristics	25.4	28.4	.01
Mother's age (years)	65.5%	34.5%	
Percent monogamous unions	42.7%	57.3%	.02
Percent polygamous unions	2.6	3.3	.05
Mother's number of children	2.5	2.9	0.1
Birth interval (years)			

An 11 x 9-inch board, one third of an inch thick and varnished of beefsteak brown colour was developed to represent a slab of meat. This meat-board was deliberately made rather large in size to convey the notion that plenty of meat was available. It was marked with a grid of lines forming 396 half-inch squares which represented pieces of meat. Mothers were asked to indicate their answers to questions about meat distribution by indicating on this board with chalk.

Questions on meat distribution

The questions investigating attitudes towards meat were as follows:

1. Imagine that you have plenty of money for food. How big a piece of meat do you think is the right amount for a two-year-old child for one meal? (show meat-board)
2. Imagine this is a piece of meat enough for one meal, and the child's father were eating with you. Please show how much meat each person in the family would get to eat. Be sure to indicate how much the two year old child will get compared to the other children. (For this second question, half of the meat-board (9" x 5.5") was used, as this was thought to represent more realistically enough meat for the entire family for one meal).
    (a) two-year-old child
    (b) mother
    (c) father
    (d) other children under five years
    (e) children between five and ten years
    (f) children between eleven and sixteen years
3. Is there any reason why you think a child of this age should not have more meat?
    (a) any more might cause child to have worms
    (b) any more might cause child to steal
    (c) any more could spoil child so he expects too much when things are scanty
4. Do you believe that giving a child of this age (two years) a lot of meat or eggs or fish could spoil his moral character?
5. Do you think a child of this age (two years) should have more meat if you can afford it?

Findings on meat distribution

In answer to question one, how big a piece of meat would be the right amount for a child of two years, the median amount of meat which mothers said they would give a two-year-old was two squares (about half a square inch). One third of the sample indicated that they would give a maximum of 1.5 or fewer squares from the meat board. Half the sample indicated a maximum of 2.5 squares or less and three quarters of the sample indicated a maximum of four squares (one square inch on the meat-board) or less.

From question two, variables were created to compute how much meat the family would eat in total for one meal, and also the percentage of this total allocated to the two-year-old child. The proportion of the family meat that would be given to the two-year-old, the median was .06. The ratio for one third of the sample was .04 or less; for two thirds of the sample .08 or less; and for three quarters .09 or less. Ninety percent of the sample showed a ratio of .11 or less, and only 3% showed a ratio of .2 or more.

In response to question three, "Is there any reason why you don't think a child of this age should have more meat?" 41% of the mothers thought that more meat might cause the child to have worms, 31% answered yes when asked if more meat might cause a child to steal, and 46% thought that giving a lot of meat would spoil the child. Most of the mothers, 66%, thought that giving more meat, eggs or fish would spoil the child's moral character, and 65% also thought a child of two should not have more meat if the family could afford it.

Trends in attitudes and practices

Table 10.11 shows the ideal amount of meat and other food investment in the child, by location. There were no statistically significant differences in these attitudes by any of the other socio-economic indicators.

There were no significant trends in the amount of meat that mothers would give, with maternal education below the level of nine years. The average amount of meat which parents with nine years of schooling or less indicated they would give their two-year-old children was three squares (three quarters of a square inch). Those mothers with an education of 10 and 11 years indicated that they would give an average amount of six squares (1.5 square inches) from the meat-board.

Table 10.11: Ideal meat portion and total food investments in the child by location

Means and ratios

Food (N=180)	Rural (N=20)	Semi-rural (N=74)	Urban (N=86)	Sig	Total
Mother's ideal meat portion for two-year-old (mean board squares)	34.3	116.5	116.8	.001	107.6
Total food investment summed weekly fruits, snacks, and animal foods excluding meat	27.3	30.0	31.6	.30	30.4
Total food investment x ideal portion size of meat	34.3	116.5	116.8	.001	107.6
Total food investment: x protein/carbohydrates, ratio	23.1	34.2	42.5	.006	36.9
Weekly meant serving x ideal portion size of meat.	1.4	4.9	3.5	.20	3.8
Ratio of meat portion for two-year-old to family total	.09	.07	.06	.01	.07

The seven mothers with 12 or more years of schooling indicated that they would give an average amount of 11 squares (2.75 square inches). On investigation it was found that the children of these seven mothers had the worst nutritional scores and the lowest average MDI scores. It is therefore probable that these women, who were relatively over-educated compared to the living standards they could afford, knew that they should be giving more meat to their growing children, but were not really doing so.

With regard to income, it was only in the top per capita income quartile that parents said that a larger quantity of meat would be given to the two-year-old (p=.10), and this is reflected in the food expenditure quartile table (Table 10.12). However, the overall proportion of the family meat given to the child did not increase, indicating that with increasing income there is no change seen in the basic attitude of the mothers.

Mothers of malnourished children were expected to give biased reports of the children's diets because of the known tendency of clinics to recommend meat for protein deficiency and fruits for diet quality. Upon examination, the mothers of children who had had kwashiorkor or marasmus were found on average to report that they would feed them slightly larger portion sizes of meat, a proportionately larger share of the family meat, slightly more frequent meat, and more frequent fruit (Table 10.13).

Associations between attitudes and practices

T-tests were used to investigate how the answers to the attitudinal questions correlated with the amount of meat a mother indicated she would give to her two-year-old child if she had no economic constraints.

Of those mothers who indicated that they would give their two-year-old child 0 to 1.5 cubes of meat, 79% believed that giving lots of meat would spoil the moral character of the child, 56% believed that giving lots of meat would spoil the child so he or she would expect too much, and 44% believed that giving lots of meat would cause the child to steal. Of those mothers who indicated that they would give their two-year-old child two to six cubes of meat, 60% believed that more would spoil the moral character of the child, 38% believed that it would give the child unrealistic expectations, and 26% believed it would cause the child to steal.

Finally, of those mothers who indicated that they would give their two-year-old the most amount of meat, 7.5 to 18 cubes from the meat-board, 44% said a lot of meat would spoil the child's moral character, 33% said meat would spoil the child so he or she expects too much, and 17% said meat would cause the child to steal.

It is clear therefore that mothers who indicated that they would give the smallest amount of meat are most likely to hold these beliefs, while those who indicated that they would give the most meat are less likely to hold such beliefs.

Practices, attitudes and nutritional status

Figure 10.1 illustrates the associations found between amounts of meat that the mother would give the two-year-old and the nutritional status of the child.

A mean difference of 0.63 SD in HAZ and 0.44 SD in WAZ favours children whose parents would give them more than 9% of the family meat compared to those who would be given less than 4%. The 0%-4% group had an average HAZ score of -2.58; the 5%-8% group, -2.22; and the 9%-22% group, -1.95, which is above the -2 SD cut-off point that delineates nutritional stunting. A similar pattern may be observed when looking at the WAZ scores, with mean values of -2.03, -1.71, and -1.61 respectively, with the highest score of 1.61 falling above the fifth percentile of the international reference standard.

Fig. 10.1: Nutritional status of child by ratio of ideal meat portion for two-year-old to family total

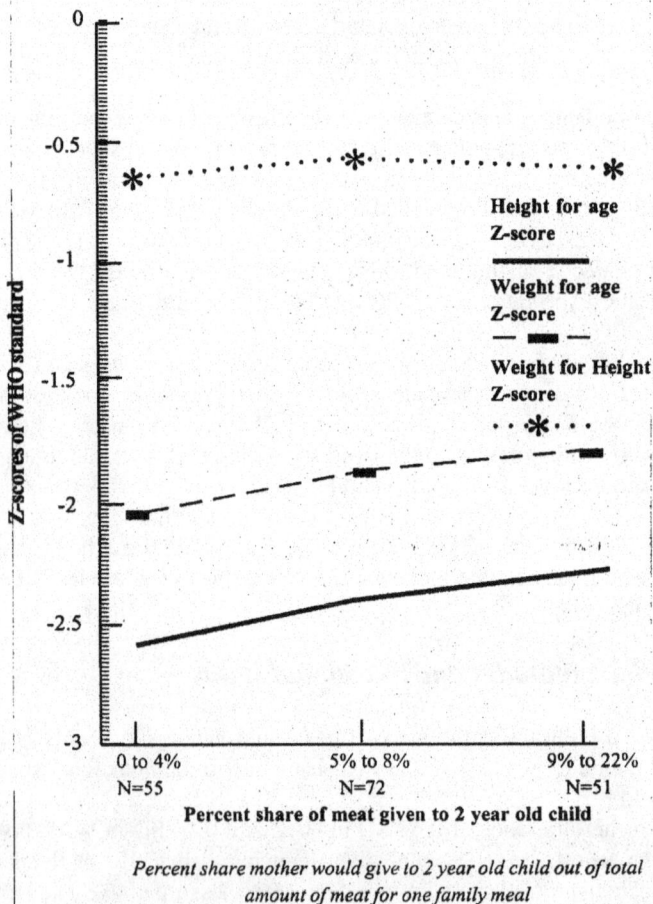

Percent share mother would give to 2 year old child out of total
amount of meat for one family meal

T-tests were used to investigate how the answers to these attitudinal questions correlated with the nutritional status, of the two-year-olds. Although none of the answers correlated significantly with the child's nutritional status, in all cases mothers with these attitudes had children whose nutritional status was lower than those whose mothers did not link meat with spoiling or stealing.

Beliefs that meat causes worms were not associated with growth. In this instance, the traditional belief that eating meat causes worms appears to some more educated parents to be a rational justification for the traditional taboos. In fact health professionals report that it is common for nurses in modern clinics to advice against giving children meat for fear of worms.

The average MDI of children whose mothers thought giving lots of meat spoils the moral character of the child was 91, while for those whose parents thought that it does not, the mean score was 95 (p<.001). In fact, the PDI (not discussed here) was the most highly associated with the belief system of all indicators. All other associations with the moral training questions were in the expected direction but at lower levels of significance.

Because only 2% of the children were acutely malnourished in terms of weight-for-height, energy does not appear to be the most limiting element in the diets of the children. Rather, our findings support the hypothesis that insufficient intake of high quality proteins and of concentrated energy in the form of oils and fats, affects concurrent cognitive function and hence is a risk factor for long term mental development.

Animal protein foods as prepared in Nigerian stews and soups provide at one time and in a single source all the essential amino acids and fatty acids for brain growth and myelinization, which involves both protein and lipid synthesis. For many but not all children, inadequacy in the supply of these nutrients leads to a rate of growth of the central nervous system which falls below the child's genetic potential during a period which is critical for the growth of the brain.

The lack of energy of the child with a poor diet also keeps him from developing cognitive skills by actively exploring and manipulating his environment and processing new information. Therefore, children who are given plenty of fish, snails, meat, eggs and other animal protein products, prepared with oil in the Nigerian manner, would experience better brain development. While bean products can substitute for animal protein products, they must also be taken in a diet prepared with sufficient oil and must be eaten more than once every day in order to do so. Thus families who give beans to the young child but do not give significant quantities of stews prepared with animal protein foods are unlikely to be able to give enough beans to make up for the lack of stew.

It may be pointed out, however, that families who can afford meat, the most costly food item, are also more likely to be able to feed their children adequately with other types of food, thus ensuring a balanced diet, and to have children who are generally better nourished. Better nourished children also tend to be healthier. They have significantly more energy and are more able to explore actively and process information from their environment, both of these advantages further stimulating their cognitive development.

The food investment variable

We hypothesized that both the frequency with which a child would be fed prestige foods and the proportional-to-seniority distribution function of the mother would impact on the development of the child. We therefore multiplied several alternative estimates of the distribution function times summary variables for the prestige foods to explore the relationships of these variables to child development.

Because of the somewhat biased relationship between reported malnutrition and the amount and reported proportions of meat given to the child, meat per se was omitted from the prestige foods summary. The distribution function for meat calculated for malnourished children was reset equal to the proportion of their individual protein-to-carbohydrate food ratios after excluding meat, times the mean value of the meat distribution variable for other not previously malnourished children.

Estimates of the distribution function included the amount the mother would give a two-year-old from Question One above, and from Question Two the two-year-old's share as a proportion of the family total, and as a proportion of the father's share. We also computed the under-fives' total as a proportion of the family total, and the two-year-old's share plus the amount for other under-fives, divided by the total under-fives as a proportion of the total.

All forms of these combined variables were much more highly correlated with nutrition and cognitive and motor scores than either the frequencies or the distribution function variables alone. The large jump in significance validated the conceptual approach of combining these two components of food investment.

Table 10.12: Ideal meat portion and total food investment in the child by food expenditure quartile and developmental group

Means and ratios

Group Food	Food expenditure quartile			Developmental		
	Low	High	Sig	Low	High	Sig
Mother's ideal meat portion for two-year-old (meat board squares)	80.8	148.8	.1	34.9	144.8	.03
Total food investment summed weekly fruits, snacks, and animal foods excluding meat	27.4	34.0	.07	26.3	31.0	.03
Total food investment x ideal portion size of meat	80.8	148.8	.1	34,8	144.8	.00
Total food investment x protein/carbohydrate ratio	30.2	44.4	.02	30.3	40.4	.01
Weekly meat serving x ideal portion size of meat	2.1	5.9	.74	3,1	4.2	.25
Ratio of meat portion for two-year-old to family total	.06	.07	.29	.07	.06	.33

The highest levels of statistical significance came from the use of the Question One amount to estimate the distribution function. This finding was expected because the question requested a simple absolute estimate ("How much is the right amount?") rather than a more complicated relative estimate.

After natural logarithmic transformation, the composite variable — right amount of meat for two-year-old multiplied by sums of weekly frequencies of snacks, fruits and animal foods not including meat.

Determinants of food investment

Table 10.13 reports the results of a regression showing determinants of the food investment variable. The most important variables are the presence of the father and a combination of the mother's education and her media exposure, followed by whether or not the mother believes that more meat would spoil the child's moral training and the age at which she introduced protein foods.

Table 10.13: Ideal meat portion and total food investment in the child by experience of kwashiorkor or marasmus

Means and ratios

	Children with K/M (N==29)	Children without (N=182)	Sig
Mother's ideal meat portion for two-year-old (meat board squares)	6.5	5.1	.71
Total food investment summed weekly fruits, snacks, and animal foods excluding meat	26.9	29.7	.21
Ideal portion size of meat	3.3	3.9	.03
Protein/carbohydrates ratio	25.4	36.8	.02
Weekly meat serving x ideal portion size of meat	3.7	3.8	.36
Ratio of meat portion for two-year-old to family total	0.08	0.07	.21

Logistic regression model

Table 10.14 reports logistic regression including the food investment variable, the eating habits variable (which combines the child having his or her own dish and eating with mother and father), the age of introducing protein foods, and the duration of breast-feeding. Among a variety of very similar and consistent models, all correctly classifying more than 95% of the children, we present only the best, together with somewhat more detailed projections of the effect sizes.

This model successfully classifies 99% of the children and has a chi-square for covariates of 101.7. It has nine independent variables for 69 cases in each developmental group, or 7.7 cases per group per variable. This ratio stretches to the limit the permissible number of variables in the equation. We consider it to be legitimate, given the stability and similarity of the models at each stage.

Table 10.14: Determinants of food investment in the child

Independent variables	Dependent variables Food investment in child*
Belief that giving meat spoils child's moral character	
B	.44
Beta	.15
Sig T	.02
Father lives with the family	
B	.36
Beta	.28
Sig T	<.001
Age of introducing protein foods	
B	-.04
Beta	.12
Sig T	<.001
Mother's media and education exposure scale	
B	-.04
Beta	.25
Sig T	.0003
Constant	2.27
Sig C	-.001
Sig F	<.001
Adjusted R2	.18
N	195

*Composite variable LINVFDI used in logarithmic form

Possibly of greatest interest is the fact that longer duration of breast-feeding emerges as a significant determinant of positive outcomes after controlling for the many other factors. Also important is the fact that rural-urban location loses significance after accounting for food investment, eating habits, and age of introducing protein foods to the children.

Discussion

The results of this study show that what mothers believe influences the way in which they feed their children; their beliefs and knowledge in turn influence the growth of the children. We conclude in this case that the environment in which people live also influences or determines what they believe.

Our sample population live in an environment in which high-quality protein foods are scarce and many people are underfed. In such conditions, there may be a strong temptation to steal what little there is for one's self. Strong social controls and moral discipline are therefore set up so that this does not occur (Agiobu-Kemmer 1989). Mothers, acting in what they think are the best interests of their children, train them to make do with very little of valued foods, or none at all, so that they will not be tempted to steal. These beliefs serve to make the child socially acceptable to the society in which he lives.

These findings also accentuate the fact that the diet of a society is influenced deeply by the cultural values placed on individual foods which are often unrelated to their nutritional value. Dietary habits affecting growth and development have social as well as economic origins, linked to value systems (Draper 1977).

At present, however, most activities including agriculture are mechanized. In order to enable children to compete in today's mechanized computer society, parents have to train their children not to become agricultural labourers on traditional farms but for a different society based on information technology and norms.

Training for the information technology age includes giving the child the types of food that would enhance this new priority, and in times of scarcity, to share with the child rather than withholding what little there is.

Table 10.15: Food investment as a predictor of low developmental group

	Odds ratio	Confidential interval	Sig
Model 1			
Intercept	100.73	.15	.16
Monogamous father	.13	.02-97	.04
Farming scale	1.76	1.15-2.67	.01
Mother's earnings per capita	9.87	2.14-45.56	<.01
Quality of child care scale	.32	.17-.61	<.01
Total child illness scale	2.46	1.27-4.77	.01
Food investment variable	.09	.02-.34	<.01
Age of introduction of protein foods	1.19	.92-1.53	.17
Eating habits variable	.33	.12-.86	.02
Duration of breastfeeding	.78	.61-1.00	.04
Chi-square for covariates	101.7		

From this survey it is known that 86% of parents want their children to attend a professional school or university, and 90% hope they will become higher-level business people or professionals. It is also evident from the results of this particular study that young children are not yet being adequately prepared for the roles to which their parents aspire for them.

Chapter 11

Nutrition and mental development

This section presents the nutritional and developmental indicators by rural and urban location and the associations between these indicators.

Nutrition and mental development by rural-urban location

The study examines the nutritional status of the children by urban, semi-rural, and rural location according to WHO standards (Lavoipierre *et al.* 1983). These standards define children who fall more than two standard deviations below the median as malnourished, as only 2.5% of children with adequate diets fall below -2 standard deviations in growth. Children who are short in height for their age (HAZ) are defined as 'stunted', while those who are too thin in weight for their height (WHZ) are termed 'wasted'.

Overall, 51% of the sample children were stunted but only 2% were wasted. This indicates that more than half of the children had adapted to inadequate diets by slowing down their growth rate and keeping their body proportions normal. The study finds that the urban children were doing better than the semi-rural and that the rural children were most seriously affected.

The study categorized the percentages malnourished according to the Gomez classification into weight-for-age categories:

third degree malnutrition = <60% of reference

median second degree   = 60-<75%
first degree   = 75%-<90%
normal   = >90%

We find that the urban children had slightly higher rates of severe malnutrition than the semi-rural, although the overall distribution of urban scores was better.

The study examined the percentages of children falling into ten-point MDI categories by location. Rural or urban location is an even stronger predictor of mental development scores than of nutritional status. As has been found in other countries (Wray), there appear to be factors associated with urbanization that lead to child stimulation of a type which enhances test scores. Of greatest interest here are the extremes: the findings that 11% of the urban, 2% of the semi-rural and none of the rural children had MDI scores above 110; while 4% of the urban, 16% of the semi-rural, and 35% of the rural scored below 80.

Table 11.1 presents the mean values and maximum and minimum scores of the nutritional indicators WAZ, HAZ, and WHZ the mental and physical development indices, MDI and PDI, and the child's mid-upper arm circumference. This table shows that rural-urban location is most strongly predictive of mental and physical development scores and show that the semi-rural and urban youngsters have very similar mean values for nutritional status.

Correlations between indicators

The Pearsons r values between the nutritional status indicators and Bayley indices are as follows:

	WAZ	HAZ	WHZ	Arm Circ	PDI
MDI	.32	.31	.18	.22	.48
PDI	.47	.47	.25	.33	

A composite measure grouping children by weight-for-height within height, as described later, had an r value of .35 with MDI.

Although all of these correlations are significant at $p<.001$, they are relatively lower values. Nutritional status explains a maximum of about 12% of the variance in MDI and 22% of the variance in PDI. These low levels of correlation confirm that some malnourished children still performed quite well, although the malnourished children as a group performed far below the well-nourished children as a group. The child with the second highest cognitive development score in the study (MDI 124) was one of the most stunted (HAZ -2.89 at 29 months). The ethnographic sub-study showed, incidentally, that this child's mother did not regularly give her any fish or meat, but fed beans to her and to her five-month-old baby sister at least once a day.

Table 11.1: Mental and physical development indices and nutritional indicators by location
Means (SD) Minimum and maximum

	Rural (N=20)	Semi-rural (N=74)	Urban (N=86)	Total (N=180)
Mental Development index				
Mean (SD)	83 (7)	94(10)	96(11)	94(11)
Minimum	69	72	77	69
Maximum	96	124	125	125
Physical development index				
Mean (SD)	99 (15)	106(14)	108(13)	196(14)
Minimum	64	79	73	64
Maximum	134	150	147	150
Height-for-age Z-score	-	-	-	-
Mean (SD)	2.58(1,05)	2.01(1,10)	2.14(1.11)	2.13(1.08)
Minimum	-4.50	-4.72	-4.35	-4.72
Maximum	-0.37	0.18	0.38	0.38
Weight-for-age Z-score	-	-	-	-
Mean (SD)	2.07(0.96)	1.54(0.88)	1.54(0.99)	1.60(0.95)
Minimum	-3.97	-3.34	-4.22	-4.22
Maximum	-0.44	1.25	0.78	1.25
Weight-for-height Z-score	-	-	-	-
Mean (SD)	0.84(0.82)	0.52(0.80)	0.38(0.81)	0.49(0.81)
Minimum	-2.21	-2.54	-2.45	-2.54
Maximum	1.16	1.62	1.53	1.62
Mid-upper arm circumference				
Mean (SD)	141(13)	144(13)	143(12)	143(12)
Minimum	116	112	111	111
Maximum	169	170	172	172

The fact that the correlation between PDI and the nutritional status variables is higher than between MDI and nutritional variables would appear to suggest that mental development is somewhat protected in a situation where malnutrition seriously delays the child's motor developmental milestones. Alternatively and perhaps more appropriately the ages of sample children being sensorimotor suggests that physical developmental milestones are a strong indication of general mental development and therefore both PDI and MDI would be quite highly correlated, but PDI would be more strongly related to nutrition as indeed they were found to be.

Mean weight-for-age shows unevenness across categories. The tallest thin group are closest in average weight-for-age (83%) to the shortest chubby group (80%).

The study also examines average MDI and PDI of the children in the six subsets. Although we cannot claim from these cross-sectional figures that malnutrition causes lasting deficits in performance, they reveal the fact that stunted chubby children were not performing as well as normally tall chubby children. In the normally tall children, average MDI was 97-98, which is quite normal and perhaps superior to the reference standard, considering the cultural bias of the Bayley test. Average PDI was 111-112, a finding consistent with the motor precocity of African children. The thinner children were not at a disadvantage when height was normal, suggesting that the thinness that expresses itself in normally tall children may reflect genetic variability or recent short-term illness in the children.

MDI and PDI decreased steadily with the degree of stunting. However, the deficits were worse among the thin stunted children than among the normally chubby ones. This finding suggests that the thinness observed in the stunted two-year-olds reflects a less adequate adaptation to nutrient insufficiency rather than a genetic difference.

Poor performers on the Bayley test and malnourished children were noted by the interviewers to have parents who were not positively attuned to them, or to be poorly attuned to their parents. The children tended to be clingy, irritable, and crying, or else withdrawn.

Some of the important findings and linkages were:

(1) There is a strong relationship between overall mental development and the children's nutritional status as measured by their height for age ($r=.32$, $p<.001$) weight for age ($r=.32$, $p<.001$) and weight for height ($r=.2$, $p<.002$).

(2) Families who eat animal protein products more frequently are more likely to have children with higher mental development ($r=.19$, $p<.003$).

(3) Children with a higher mental development index (MDI) are those to whom the mother would be willing to give a larger amount of meat per meal if a plentiful supply were available.

(4) The size of the meat portion given to the two-year-old at one meal which appears to be associated with a higher overall mental development is about 3.5 cubic inches. Two-year-old children who obtained this amount or more tended to have significantly higher mental development.

Discussion

As noted in the introduction to this study, we cannot attempt to generalize concerning the size of the relationship between malnutrition and mental development. We wish, however, to underscore the invisibility and complexity of the problem.

The invisibility of the problem

The average stunted two-year-old child is both nutritionally compromised and cognitively at risk as indicated by low test scores. Yet it is not possible to detect the majority of these children by any visible signs. Stunted children look normal. They do not look malnourished, except perhaps for the presence of a pot belly, which can be an indication that the body has adapted to inadequate food. Adipose tissue on the abdomen may metabolically maintain normal blood sugar levels and assist in slowing down the rate of growth, in order to keep the amount of all nutrients circulating in the blood supply adequate for the body's day-to-day operations. (See pp. 29-32 in Zeitlin *et al.*, 1990)

The 2% of children who are truly wasted are poorly adapted to food insufficiency, often because they have recently been ill. Except for the rare cases of kwashiorkor, these thin children are the only ones who are visibly malnourished. Therefore, only about 5% of malnutrition and associated low performance can be seen. Most of the loss to the children is invisible.

Chapter 12

Interactional aspects of childcare

A major purpose of this study was to obtain detailed information regarding the quality of child care, with respect to the mother-child interaction and the richness of experience available in the child's environment.

In addition to the Bayley Scales of Infant Development, two psychological tests were administered:

(1) A set of behaviour and affect ratings (Cravioto and Pericardie, 1976) completed by the interviewer who administered the Bayley test, based on her reactions to the mother and child during the test situation.

(2) The Caldwell and Bradley (1984) Home Observation for the Measurement of the Environment (HOME) Inventory.

The behaviour and affect ratings and the Caldwell HOME inventory were designed primarily to predict IQ and other psychological test performance in North American settings. Our use of these tests differs from this original intent to the extent that we examined associations with our combined developmental measure and with growth status. We also investigated associations with the Bayley scores. However, because of the cultural differences between our sample and the reference population, our investigation was primarily exploratory.

Behaviour and affect ratings

The Behaviour and Affect Ratings record the Bayley tester's assessment of:

(a) Mother's behaviour and affect,

(b) Infant behaviour and affect,
(c) Examiner reactions to the child and the mother during testing.

All items are rated on a five point scale (1-5). Training was done in small groups in the homes, while inter-observer reliability was established in the classroom setting on four children with scores above 80.

Rural-urban trends

Tables 12.1 to 12.3 display the three sets of scale items contrasted by location. Unless otherwise indicated, these tables give percentages rated above average (scores of 4 or 5) on each item.

The rural mothers were significantly more likely to urge their children to do the Bayley test with scolding, teasing and threats (Table 12.1). A difference between the rural children and the rest of the sample commented upon by all of the interviewers at debriefing was their shyness and clinginess to their mothers (Table 12.2). The rural children were judged significantly less eager and joyful, more difficult for the interviewer to elicit a positive affective response from, and more withdrawn or emotionally averted.

The interviewers were significantly more likely to respond to the rural mothers with a negative reaction of anger, dislike or avoidance, and somewhat more likely to judge them as less joyful, comforting and emotionally available. (Table 12.3) The interviewers also found the urban children more attractive, and easier to elicit task-oriented behaviour and positive responses from.

Factor analysis revealed underlying dimensions in the behaviour and affect ratings which were used to group the variables into the following composite measures:
(1) Co-operative child: perceived by examiner as easy to test; well synchronized with interviewer; easy to elicit positive affect and task-oriented behaviour from; not angry, irritable, provocative, withholding, averting or intrusive; and not eliciting a negative response from the tester.
(2) Skilled mother: managing the child well; and not disruptive, intrusive or over-controlling.
(3) Eliciting child: eager or joyful; with a gleam in the eye; appealing and attractive; and eliciting an examiner reaction of falling in love with the child, wanting to touch or cuddle the child.

Table 12.1: Behaviour and affect rating of mother by location

Percentages

	Rural (N=20)	Semi-rural (N=74)	Urban (N=86)	Total (N=180)
Is eager, joyful	55%	72%	66%	68%
Encourages with positive reinforcement	60%	61%	57%	59%
Urges with scolding, teasing, threats	35%	10%	7%	11%
Shows visible pleasure in child's achievement	60%	70%	65%	67%
Is not visibly upset by child's failure	35%	41%	44%	42%
Attempts to guide child	80%	74%	71%	73%
Manages child well	40%	63%	60%	59%
Disrupts child's activities	15%	8%	11%	10%
Expresses hostility	5%	12%	6%	8%
Comforts child, or expresses approval, affection	40%	52%	59%	54%
Never tunes out or withdraw emotionally from child	20%	23%	21%	22%
Emotionally available, warm, rewarding, responsive	65%	75%	77%	75%
Empathically responsive	65%	68%	65%	66%

Table 12.2: Behaviour and affect rating of child by location

Percentages

	Rural (N=20)	Semi-rural (N=74)	Urban (N=86)	Total (N=180)
Flat, placid, no eagerness	45%	23%	18%	24%
Irritable, distressed	35%	28%	4%	26%
No anger or aggression (lowest score)	20%	33%	33%	32%
Shows provocative teasing, testing	40%	23%	20%	23%
Emotionally withdraw, averted	50%	26%	18%	25%
Ra t her or very withholding	45%	27%	26%	28%
Never intrusive or grabby (lowest score)	15%	32%	31%	30%
Reciprocal, well synchronized with tester	10%	53%	48%	49%
Has gleam in eyes	25%	55%	48%	49%
Appealing and attractive child	40%	50%	55%	51%

(4) Warm rewarding mother: comforting, encouraging, eager or joyful; visibly pleased with the child's performance; not withdrawn from the child; emotionally rewarding, empathetic; and attractive or appealing to the interviewer.

(5) Critical mother: expressing hostility or sarcasm; urging performance with scolding, teasing, or threats; and visibly upset or disappointed by the child's failure.

(6) Needy mother: eliciting dislike or nurturing feelings in the tester, as if the mother were needy or immature.

Table 12.4 shows that the rural children were found to be significantly less eliciting and co-operative, and their mothers to be significantly more often perceived by the interviewers as "needy."

Table 12.3: Tester's reactions to mother and child by location

Percentages

	Rural (N=20)	Semi-rural (N=74)	Urban (N=86)	Total (N=180)
Mother				
Tester found mother attractive, appealing	45%	61%	65%	61%
Tester felt nurturing towards mother as if she were young or immature (average or higher score)	30%	16%	14%	17%
Tester reacted negatively to mother, was angered, disliked or avoided (average or higher score)	25%	4%	6%	7%
Child				
Tester found it easy to elicit positive affective response	30%	54%	59%	54%
Tester found it easy to elicit task-oriented behaviour	35%	47%	58%	51%
Tester attracted to child	25%	40%	38%	38%
Tester had negative response to child	25%	27%	18%	23%

Rural-urban differences

Although close to the metropolitan area, the rural site was hidden, away from the road and "back woods" in character. A clash of values and lifestyles appeared to contribute to perceived urban-rural differences, affecting responses of both the adults and children.

The good mother according to traditional child-rearing norms engages in more obedience training and less rewarding and stimulating interaction. The rural mothers might have tended to view the test as a set of chores that an obedient child should be able to do. The rural two-year-olds not only lacked exposure to urban dress, assertive styles of speech, and toys, and also showed a tendency of not wanting to engage in technical play with the testing toys. The interviewers, all psychology graduates of the University of Lagos, were emotionally invested in promoting a more modern interactive style of child rearing, and hence likely to view these rural children more negatively.

Table 12.4: Behaviour and affect scales by location

	Means			
	Rural (N=20)	Semi-rural (N=74)	Urban (N=86)	Total (N=180)
Cooperative child	2.0	2.5	2.6	2.5
Skilled mother	3.75	3.9	3.8	3.9
Eliciting child	2.9	3.3	3.4	3.3
Warm rewarding mother	3.4	3.7	3.6	3.6
Critical mother	2.5	2.3	2.3	2.3

Differences in behaviour and affect by developmental group

Tables 12.5 and 12.6 give those ratings on which the testers' perceptions of the mothers and children differed significantly by developmental group. Mothers of the high group were less likely to guide or disrupt, better able to manage the child, and more emotionally available. High group children were more eager and joyful, and less irritable, angry, provocative, withdrawn, or intrusive, being more co-operative overall.

Tester reactions and scale scores in Table 12.7 show that the examiners found the high group children significantly more attractive and eliciting.

For this set of variables, however, contrasts based only on the composite developmental score mask important differences between correlates of nutritional status and correlates of cognitive test performance. Variables on the maternal warmth/rewarding and co-operative baby scales are highly correlated to developmental test scores but uncorrelated or only marginally related to nutritional status.

Specifically the following variables were found to be significant with the MDI but showed no association to nutrition; for the mother: emotionally withdrawn, and emotionally available during the test; for the child: angry, provocative, intrusive, easy to elicit positive affective and task-oriented responses from, and whether the interviewer had a negative response to the child. The critical mother scale was significant and negative with MDI but marginally positive with HAZ.

Table 12.5: Behaviour and affect ratings of mother by developmental group

	Low (N=69)	High (N=69)
Attempts to guide child	83%	67%
Manages child well (highest score)	6%	17%
Never disrupts child's activities (lowest score)	20%	33%
Never withdraws emotionally from child (lowest score)	20%	33%
Is highly emotionally available to child	9%	16%

Implications of differences in behaviour and affect by developmental group

The differences noted between malnutrition and test score correlates may be expected in that malnutrition creates a less active and hence more compliant and weaker child, appearing more in need of nurturance. Well nourished two-year-olds are extremely active and often provocative, and so potentially more likely to elicit maternal control, withdrawal or criticism. Because better nourished children are, by definition, bigger and are more advanced in their behaviour, they are perceived to be more mature and are hence subject to more task training and discipline.

Table 12.6: Behaviour and affect ratings of child by developmental group

Percentages

	Low (N=69)	High (N=69)
Flat, placid, no eagerness (below average)	35%	13%
Eager, joyful (highest score)	4%	19%
No anger or aggression (lowest score)	23%	41%
Often aggressive or angry	28%	16%
No provocative behaviours (lowest score)	13%	32%
Not emotionally withdrawn or averted	48%	70%
Never intrusive, grabby (lowest score)	26%	41%
Reciprocal, well synchronized with tester	26%	68%
Has gleam in eyes	41%	65%
Appealing and attractive child	38%	61%

Malnutrition causes children to be irritable and lacking in joy and "gleam in the eyes," yet may be associated with greater compliance with adult demands. In this population, the same child-rearing code which restricts food for the child actively trains him in obedience and social responsiveness. Not surprisingly, 51% of the lowest and 48% of the highest WAZ tertile children were judged easy to elicit task-oriented behaviour from, and 15% of the lowest versus 13% of the highest evoked no negative response from the tester.

Table 12.7: Tester's reactions to mother and child by developmental group

Percentages

	Low (N=69)	High (N=69)
Mother		
Tester found mother attractive, appealing	57%	70%
Tester felt nurturing towards mother as if she were young or immature (average or higher score)	19%	9%
Tester reacted negatively to mother, was angered, disliked or avoided (average or higher score)	12%	1%
Child		
Tester found it easy to elicit positive affective response	43%	71%

	Low (N=69)	High (N=69)
Tester found it easy to elicit task-oriented behaviour	45%	64%
Tester attracted to child	23%	48%
Tester had negative response to child	30%	13%

Well-nourished children were rated by the testers (who were unaware of their nutritional status) as more eager and reciprocal in their behaviour than malnourished children (r=.18, p<.004). Malnourished children appeared dull, unattractive and less likely to stimulate adults' interactive response (r=.16, p<.01). Children with higher weight-for-height Z-scores had parents who scored higher in the Parental Involvement scale (r=.13, p<.05) and Provision of Play Materials scale (r=.13, p<.05) of the HOME Inventory. These findings are consistent with data from other studies (e.g. Barret, 1984; Dasen *et al..*, 1977).

These findings imply that the malnourished children are deprived of the stimulation and learning experiences which interactions with their mothers could facilitate during this critical period of their development. It is therefore not surprising that their mental development is delayed.

Evidence for child-driven outcomes

Table 12.8 gives behaviour and affect scales by developmental group. The eliciting-child scale has highly significant positive correlations with all of the nutritional status and developmental indicators, with the food investment variable and with the belief that it is not necessary to withhold meat for the child's moral training. Also, the co-operative child scale is highly correlated to food investment and to the belief that giving meat will not cause the child to steal, while the mother who is highly critical of her child is more likely to believe that giving meat would cause him to steal. These associations are consistent with the work of other researchers (Caldwell and Bradley 1984) and a general consensus that the child's own characteristics influence the parents' response.

The relative strength of these associations points to the conclusion that under conditions of scarcity, a child's attractiveness may greatly influence his or her access to high quality foods and attention, and hence the developmental outcome. A child that appears to the field worker to be unattractive may be a child at high risk, as physical signs of severe malnutrition in the child have been found to trigger emotional abandonment by the mother.

Table 12.8: Behaviour and affect scales by developmental group

Means (SD)

	Low (N=69)	High (N=69)	Sig
Cooperative child	2.29(.84)	2.72(.86)	.0024
Skilled mother	3.66(.85)	3.99(.77)	.034
Eliciting child	3.01(.78)	3.58(.83)	.0001
Warm, rewarding mother	3.60(.56)	3.74(.55)	.09
Critical mother	2.35(.72)	2.30(.64)	.92

Cultural distance associations

Rural-urban differences in adherence to traditional cultural parenting norms might be reflected in maternal behaviours more consistent with obedience training than with stimulating interaction. We hypothesized that other measures of cultural distance, such as the farming scale and the food investment variable, would show similar associations with the behaviour and affect ratings. In fact, mothers high on the warm rewarding scale also scored significantly higher on the food investment variable and significantly lower on ties to farming. Mothers who believed that more meat would not spoil the child's moral character were marginally more likely (p=.11) to be judged as rewarding.

Caldwell and Bradley's HOME Inventory

The Caldwell Home Observation for Measurement of the Environment, commonly referred to as the HOME Inventory (Caldwell and Bradley 1984) was developed to sample the quality and quantity of social, emotional and cognitive support available to the young child in his home environment. It attempts to determine those aspects of the home environment which are most important in predicting a child's later developmental outcomes.

The test, conducted partly by observation and partly by interview, comprises six subscales:

  I.   Emotional and verbal responsivity
  II.   Acceptance of the child's behaviour
  III. Organization of the environment

IV.   Provision of play materials
V.   Parental involvement
VI.   Opportunity for variety of stimulation

We selected the widely applied HOME Inventory for the Nigerian study because it had been used in our Indonesian study, thereby offering an opportunity for cross-cultural comparison, and because it had previously been found to predict malnutrition in a developing country environment (Cravioto 1972).

It was necessary to adapt this test both to suit the period over which the two field workers were present in each home, and to the levels of poverty in the homes. Our time window, which was longer than the normal administration time for the HOME, gave more opportunity for the mother to be observed interacting with the child through talking, caressing, etc. The administration of the Bayley test during this time also created an opportunity for observing atypical mother-child interactions. For example when the mother might be more likely than usual, to label test objects for the child, who might be sitting on her lap.

Adaptations included replacing certain yes/no categories with never, sometimes, and usually variables or with counts of objects or occurrences, with a view to finding meaningful cut-points in the data during analysis. We embedded the HOME items into a naturally flowing sequence within the socioeconomic status/mother questionnaire. The field worker who did not administer the Bayley administered the HOME subscales as part of this questionnaire.

A few questions were also culturally adapted, due to the cultural differences between Nigeria and North America and the expectation we expected that the Caldwell items and scales would perform differently in the two populations.

While relatively thematically consistent, the scales of the Caldwell were assembled on the basis of factor analysis, leading to inclusion of some apparently unrelated items in various scales. For example, "Parent permits child to engage in messy play," is in the Emotional and Verbal Responsivity scale; and "At least 10 books are present and visible," is in the Acceptance of Child's Behaviour scale.

Hypotheses

Based on the cross-cultural literature on parenting (e.g. LeVine, 1974, LeVine *et al.*, 1988; Scheper-Hughes, 1987), we viewed parenting codes as compromise formulas for preparing children for their adult roles, while protecting them from risks in the child care environment. We hypothesized three layers of relationship:

(1) Variables designed to measure parental values in the reference culture which do not exist in a second culture will tend not to predict developmental outcomes in that second culture. When this lack of prediction occurs, it will indicate that the behaviours being measured are relevant to the desired outcomes only in the value system of the culture in which the test was designed and not in the second culture in which it is administered.

Conversely, sets of variables capturing parental values in the second culture which do not exist in the first will predict developmental outcomes in the second culture, but not the first.

(2) Parents who are conscientious in applying the codes of their culture will have better child outcomes than parents who are incompetent or indifferent in applying those codes. To some degree this relationship will be seen even when differences in cultural codes lead to seemingly contradictory types of behaviour in different cultures, and even when the culturally encoded behaviours do not directly foster the outcomes measured.

Parents whose behaviours reflect adherence to more modern codes will have children whose developmental status conforms more closely to the modern performance standards reflected in our measurements of growth status and cognitive scores.

(3) Children perceived as particularly vulnerable will receive more nurturing treatment to reduce their susceptibility to risk. This effect will be prominent in cultures with high infant mortality (LeVine *et al.*, 1990), and will be confounding. It will reduce the significance of all associations, because the households who would otherwise score lowest on the HOME will have the sickest and most malnourished children who may receive extra compensatory attention.

Basic to the above hypotheses and the cultural theories underlying them is that the adaptiveness of given parenting behaviours depends on the environmental living conditions and resources available.

We however, first reviewed the original HOME scales and items for children from birth to three years before examining our research results.

Values differing in Nigerian and reference cultures

One value stronger in the North American reference culture than in Nigerian culture is acceptance of child's behaviour, meaning the child's independence or autonomy, which is measured in Scale II. As shown by

Hoffman (1988) in an eight-country cross-national study, independence in children is of greater value to North Americans than it is to most Asians. The study also showed that within countries, parents of farmers and manual and service workers tended to place a higher value on obedience than independence when compared to professional and skilled and clerical workers. Caldwell and Bradley (1984) report that the acceptance scale was less relevant to outcomes among black than white Americans. In accord with the first hypothesis, we did not expect to see a positive relationship between outcomes in Nigerian children and Scale II.

A part of the child-rearing code for children of this age in Nigerian culture is the value placed upon didactic teaching. Caldwell (1968) lists the 12 characteristics of developmentally stimulating environments on which the HOME is based. Notably absent from this list is any didactic teaching of the child under three years. The absence of didactic items in the 0-3 Bayley may also be primarily a matter of convenience, as it would be impossible to have didactic activities that were appropriate across the 0-3 age range. By contrast, however, traditional Yoruba culture has started to teach the two-year-old some chores and tasks, and 69% of our sample mothers claimed to actively teach the ABC's.

A second characteristic Nigerian value is the socialization of the young child for lifelong contribution to the immediate and extended family. As indicated in Chapter 4, this socialization among the Yoruba requires the child to accept a role subordinate to his seniors, rather than a companionship role. The subordinate role may require the child not to speak in front of strangers unless cued to do so by a superior. Parenting behaviours that reflect skill in creating a cheerful and respectful subordinate child by Nigerian standards would not be measured by the HOME inventory.

The Nigerian study population, in which 70% of families shared a single room usually face-to-face across a narrow corridor from the room shared by another family, lived in far more crowded circumstances than in the reference population. Some of the 12 characteristics of developmentally stimulating environments appeared likely to be violated by these crowded conditions.

Review of HOME inventory scales

In applying the different component scales of the HOME inventory, beginning with Scale I, Emotional and Verbal Responsivity, to our Nigerian sample, we did not expect to find strong associations of developmental outcomes with praise or verbal indications of approval.

These might be feared to be overly expressive in front of strangers, to spoil the child or to invoke supernatural ill fortune. We expected rather that the cultural environment was so structured that complete but attentive silence might be even more rewarding to the child's performance than vocalization. Permitting the child to engage in "messy" play did not seem a likely relevant expression of responsivity in the Nigerian context.

In Scale II, it was hypothesized that shouting, annoyance and physical punishment were more likely to be meted out by conscientious mothers to active well-nourished children. Item II-15, on physical punishment, had to be modified to reflect more frequent cuffing (often by flicking with the mother's finger tips joined together) than in the reference population. Ten books (Item II-18) were beyond the reach of most homes, and dogs and cats tended to be work animals rather than pets, therefore not evoking the same empathy and anthropomorphizing or role-playing behaviours as in the reference group.

The crowding in low-income Nigerian homes and neighbourhoods virtually ensured that the children got "out of the house" and often visited with relatives (Scales III and VI). The benefit of such outings (III-21 and 22) is confounded by the fact that the children who visited the most places tended to be those taken to work by mothers who had no other child care arrangements for them.

In Scale IV, several of the items refer to types of toys that provide learning opportunities for specific aspects of motor co-ordination. Items 30 and 34 investigated toys facilitating dramatic or social play (as also do the motor toys). Only Item 33 (and to a lesser extent 31) could be considered specific to the technical play for which Nigerian children have been found to have fewer opportunities than western children (Whiten and Milner, 1984; Agiobu-Kemmer, 1984).

Since the Nigerian two-year-olds scored higher in motor skills than the reference group but had very few motor toys, with the exception of balls, we did not feel that presence of the different types of motor toys *per se* would have much relevance to development in the Nigerian sample. The Nigerian child's participation in dancing might have been more relevant to motor co-ordination. Nevertheless, the presence of purchased toys would reflect the parents' investment in the child and the parents' grasp of the concept that children learn through play, thereby dignifying the child's play activities with approval and participation.

Before creating the questionnaire section on toys and play objects, we conducted a toy inventory, of purchased, home-made, and improvised toys and play materials in a low- income neighbourhood adjacent to the University of Lagos.

Given the low number of toys available in the households, we introduced the presentation of a book during the home visit in order to measure Scale V, item 38.

With respect to Scale VI, the father's presence in the home too is important to the child but most probably for instrumental reasons rather than as a source of "variety" alone. Similarly, the child's eating with both parents was found to be positively associated with development, but probably as an indicator of modern monogamous family lifestyle, not for reasons of "variety".

HOME Inventory variables by location

Before looking for rural-urban trends in the HOME scales, it is worth noting major characteristics of the population.

The high level of social interaction with the children seen in the ethnographic study was confirmed by the 97% of mothers reporting social play with the child and the 92% of children playing with their fathers or another adult male daily. In rates almost as high, 95% of children possessed a "pretend" and 18% a real musical instrument. Virtually all Yoruba children engage in drumming and dancing. Songs and verses and the *oriki* were recited to 87%. The *oriki* is a poetic genealogy or praise name, specially composed to honour the individuality and destiny of each child. The ethnographic study also records singing by the children and their families.

Task training had started for 99% of the two-year-olds who helped their mothers by taking "things from one place to another;" 97% were learning to carry water in a small bowl; 93% to wash their own hands or face; and 93% to put their own things away. An astonishing number of two-year-olds (75%) were already sent on errands to buy things, as also observed in the ethnographic study, while 39% could wash their own plate or cup and 28% already were learning housework chores such as sweeping, washing clothes, etc.

Motivation for academic success was extremely high. Of those children who had older siblings, 78% had siblings who were attending "lessons" or privately paid coaching sessions above and beyond conventional school attendance. Overall 58% of mothers claimed to be already preparing the two-year-old for school and 69%, as noted earlier, to be teaching the child ABC's and 1,2,3.

The concern for academic success is consistent with the high percentage of parents aspiring for their children to become professionals as shown by location in Table 12.9. These aspirations were not used for further analysis because the ethnography indicated that less educated and aware mothers tended to have more unrealistically high aspirations for their children than mothers of high scorers, who more realistically assessed their children's prospects.

Despite these widely shared characteristics, rural-urban differences on the HOME scale also appeared, reflected in Tables 12.10 to 12.16. Rural mothers were less likely to respond verbally to the child's verbalizations, to tell the child the name of an object, or to start a conversation with the field worker (Table 12.10). They were also less likely to shout or express hostility towards the child, although more likely to say the child required spanking so many times a day that they could not remember exactly (Table 12.11). Rural and semi-rural children went less frequently to the market and shops, although they more often visited the houses of relatives and friends (Table 12.12).

Table 12.9: Mother's aspirations for child by location

	Rural (N=20)	Semi-rural (N=74)	Urban (N=86)	Total (N=180)
Desired level of education to be achieved by child				
High School	25%	10%	5%	9%
Post secondary, polytechnic, college of education	5%	6%	4%	5%
University or professional school	70%	85%	92%	86%
Desirable job or occupation for child after finishing school				
Skilled labourer, craftsperson, carpenter, soldier, policeman	20%	6%	5%	7%
Taxi driver	5%	1%	0%	2%
Clerical	5%	3%	1%	4%
Minister, priest, imam, babalawo	5%	0%	0%	1%
Higher level shopkeeper of business person	30%	33%	40%	36%
Professional	35%	57%	54%	54%

There was a rural-urban gradient in the number of types of books and visual materials visible in the homes, and in the total number of books and school books in the home (Tables 12.11 and 12.16). Ownership of books by the child was reported to be higher in the small rural sample (Table 12.15). This finding, which was undoubtedly atypical of rural areas more generally, probably stemmed from some circumstance, such as proselytizing by an Adventist group that had distributed books or pamphlets in the rural sample location. The urban children were more likely to have their own chair or bed (Table 12.13) and a place to keep their toys or treasures (Table 12.12). Both variety of manufactured toys and total number owned increased progressively with urbanization (Tables 12.13 and 12.16).

Table 12.10: Mother's emotional and verbal responsivity by location

	Rural (N=20)	Semi-rural (N=74)	Urban (N=86)	Total (N=180)
I-1 Number of times mother spontaneously spoke to the child				
None	35%	43%	48%	44%
One	15%	11%	12%	12%
Two	25%	20%	14%	18%
Three or more	25%	26%	27%	26%
I-2 Mother's verbal response to child's verbalizations				
Made non-verbal sounds				
Never	80%	92%	86%	88%
Sometimes	15%	5%	8%	8%
Usually	5%	3%	6%	5%
Used simple words the child could repeat				
Never	55%	50%	47%	49%
Sometimes	35%	35%	44%	39%
Usually	10%	15%	9%	12%
Used adult speech				
Never	20%	10%	8%	10%
Sometimes	65%	38%	35%	56%
Usually	15%	53%	57%	43%
I-3 Told the child the name of an object				
Never	0%	1%	1%	1%
Sometimes	35%	57%	61%	56%
Usually	65%	42%	38%	43%
I-4 Speech was audible and clear	95%	97%	98%	97%
I-5 Started a conversation with field workers	10%	27%	32%	28%
I-6 Conversed freely and easily with field workers	90%	87%	94%	91%
I-7 Let the child play with "messy" mud, water, sand	22%	10%	13%	13%
I-8 Spontaneously praised child at least twice	55%	35%	51%	45%

	Rural (N=20)	Semi-rural (N=74)	Urban (N=86)	Total (N=180)
I-9 Conveyed positive feelings toward child by tone of voice	85%	81%	87%	84%
I-10 Caressed or kissed child at least once	50%	54%	50%	52%
I-11 Responded positively to praise of child	30%	30%	28%	29%

Didactic teaching to prepare the two-year-old for school was much more common among urban mothers (Table 12.14), as was the attendance of an older sibling at "lessons" (Table 12.15). Story telling to the child, and recitation of songs and verses, traditional rural "by moonlight" activities were more commonly reported by urban mothers (Table 12.15).

The urban mothers were most engaged in teaching the children to do chores such as sweeping and washing dishes, and also had the highest rates of teaching self-help skills such as washing one's own hands and face. These aspects of socialization and investment in the child appear in Table 12.16.

Table 12.11: Mother's acceptance of child's behaviour HOME Scale II by location

Means (SD) and percentages

	Rural (N=20)	Semi-rural (N=74)	Urban (N=86)	Total (N=180)
II-12 Shouted at child	15%	23%	17%	20%
II-13 Expressed annoyance or hostility	20%	13%	9%	12%
II-14 Slapped or spanked child	10%	7%	12%	9%
II-15 Said child does not usually obey, requires punishment	20%	23%	18%	20%
Said child needed spanking				
Never	25%	13%	18%	20%
More than once a week, but less than daily	55%	80%	76%	75%
Many times a week, can't remember exactly	20%	7%	6%	8%
II-16 Scolds or criticizes the child	10%	16%	14%	14%
II-17 Did not interfere with or restrict the child more than three time	0%	1%	0%	1%
II-18 Visual reading or teaching materials in home				
Number of books in home	3(2.1)	4(2.1)	4(2.2)	4(2.2)

	Rural (N=20)	Semi-rural (N=74)	Urban (N=86)	Total (N=180)
Picture books	30%	35%	57%	45%
Story books	15%	37%	48%	40%
Picture calendars	45%	85%	86%	81%
Magazines with pictures	15%	45%	59%	50%
Older child's school books	55%	62%	73%	67%
School notebooks	55%	57%	69%	63%
Il-19 Pet-cat or dog in home				
None	75%	76%	76%	76%
Present, child not allowed to play with it	0%	3%	8%	5%
Present, child allowed to play with it.	25%	22%	16%	19%

HOME inventory variables by developmental group

Tables showing the HOME variables by developmental group include, in addition to statistically significant contrasts, key variables which although hypothesized to differ by group showed no significant differences.

In this test setting, the mothers' frequency of spontaneous speech to the child did not differ by group, although high-group children were more likely to have mothers who responded to their vocalizations with simple words or nonsense sounds than with adult speech or not at all (Table 12.17). High group mothers were also more likely to converse freely and easily with the field workers. The ethnographic study described marked differences in quality and quantity of verbal interchange between families of high and low scorers; talkativeness of both mothers and children was seen in the top group.

As expected, spontaneous praise and caressing rates were marginally higher for low-group children, while shouting, hostility, slapping, and criticism were higher in the high group (Table 12.18), possibly because more high-group mothers claimed that their children did not "usually obey."

There was almost no difference in percentages having a special place to keep toys or treasures (Table 12.18). More high-group children had their own beds and chairs, but marginally more of the low group had their own cup, plate or spoon (Table 12.19), possibly because the family did not own complete place settings for all household members. The high group had more self-help skills (hand and face-washing and putting their own things away) but performed about the same number of household chores (Tables 12.21 and 12.23).

Table 12.12: Organization of the environment HOME Scale II by location

Percentages

	Rural (N=20)	Semi-rural (N=74)	Urban (N=86)	Total (N=180)
III-20 Child has 1-3 primary caretakers	44%	54%	62%	55%
III-21 Child accompanies mother every week to:				
Market	0%	0%	27%	28%
Shops	10%	36%	43%	36%
Church	50%	54%	69%	60%
Mosque	18%	19%	21%	19%
House of relatives	50%	43%	28%	37%
House of friends	45%	30%	24%	29%
III-22 Child usually accompanies mother to work	44%	54%	62%	55%
Total number of outings per week child accompanies mother				
0	10%	10%	9%	9%
1-2	60%	45%	46%	47%
3-4	25%	28%	32%	30%
5-6	5%	16%	14%	14%
III-23 Number of times child taken for check-up when not ill				
0-7	90%	76%	73%	76%
≥8	10%	24%	27%	24%
III-24 Child has special place to keep toys or treasures	25%	27%	38%	32%
III-25 Child's play environment is safe	60%	75%	66%	69%

High-group children had significantly more manufactured toys, and total picture books, school books and notebooks visible in the home, but fewer improvised toys (Table 12.20). Their mothers were more likely to teach them "ABC, 123", and to engage with them in technical play or socio-technical play rather than social play alone (Table 12.21). More than twice as many high group children (68% vs. 33%) had someone read to them from books. There was non-significantly more attendance at coaching sessions by high-group siblings and by the children themselves (Table 12.22). Investment in toys and books and teaching of self-help skills were all higher in the high group (Table 12.23).

Significantly more high-group children ate with their mothers and fathers together at least three times in a week, and more played with their father or another adult male daily.

Table 12.13: Provision of play materials Home Scale IV by location

Percentages

	Rural (N=20)	Semi-rural (N=74)	Urban (N=86)	Total (N=180)
IV-31 Child has own:				
Cup, plate, or spoon	80%	69%	78%	74%
Chair	45%	45%	65%	54%
Crib, or bed	5%	8%	13%	10%
IV-32 Manufactured toys				
Football	15%	11%	14%	13%
Plastic ball	0%	12%	7%	8%
Wheeled toy to sit on	5%	8%	4%	6%
Rocking horse	5%	4%	6%	5%
Toy car	5%	3%	7%	5%
Toy plane	0%	1%	1%	1%
Wind-up toy	0%	0%	1%	1%
Plastic doll	30%	16%	20%	20%
Plastic rattle	15%	5%	14%	11%
Blocks	0%	0%	0%	0%
Plastic building toys "legos"	0%	1%	0%	1%
Puzzles	0%	0%	0%	0%
Crayons	0%	0%	0%	0%
Real or toy musical instrument	15%	15%	21%	18%
Teddy bear, other stuffed animal	0%	0%	2%	1%
Other toys	5%	11%	20%	15%
IV-33 Homemade toys				
Bottle covers	15%	15%	31%	22%
Special stones, sticks	20%	24%	22%	23%
Empty tins	55%	65%	41%	53%
Plastic cups, other plastic containers	5%	34%	22%	25%
School box	0%	5%	1%	3%
Paper or newspaper	0%	7%	15%	10%
Plastic bag	15%	12%	11%	12%
Special cloth	0%	7%	6%	6%
Pretend musical instrument	100%	91%	98%	95%
Sand or mud	35%	38%	19%	29%
Water	5%	17%	15%	15%
Games	20%	30%	24%	26%

Construction of the established HOME scales

For the purpose of cross-cultural comparison, the established HOME scales were constructed from the HOME variables. For this purpose, variables with more than one response category were recoded to binary variables, used in the HOME, at the break-points that captured variability in the population. As an exception, variables intended to be virtually constant for children living in normal homes (Caldwell and Bradley 1984) were not recoded.

The results in Table 12.24 show that the Nigerian children's scores on the HOME subscales were comparable to those of the Caldwell and Bradley (1984) twenty-four-month-old sample, with the exception of the Organization of the Environment and the Provision of Play Materials subscales. Correlation analyses of these subscales with the children's performance on the Bayley Tests did not yield meaningful results. The HOME subscales were therefore not very useful as instruments for measuring the salient aspects of the home environment as related to the sample infants, cognitive functioning. Table 12.25 shows very low reliability coefficients for the scales compared with Caldwell's results for the same scales.

Table 12.14: Parental involvement Home Scale V by location

Percentages

	Rural (N=20)	Semi-rural (N=74)	Urban (N=86)	Total (N=180)
V-35 Mother keeps child in visual range, looks at often	65%	63%	80%	72%
Mother plays with child	95%	97%	100%	98%
Engages in social play	95%	99%	97%	97%
Technical lay with toys or objects	11%	3%	17%	11%
Socio-technical play, including social interaction and objects	32%	25%	29%	27%
V-36 Parent talks to child while doing housework				
Never	35%	43%	48%	44%
Once	15%	11%	12%	12%
Twice	25%	20%	14%	18%
Three or more times	25%	26%	27%	26%
V-37 Has taught child to:				
Take tings from one place to another	95%	100%	100%	99%
Carry water in a small bowl	95%	97%	97%	97%
Wash own plate or cup	35%	38%	41%	39%
Put own tings away	90%	90%	95%	93%
Buy things	70%	74%	78%	75%
Do housework (e.g. sweeping, washing clothes)	10%	37%	25%	28%
Number of different chores performed by child				
None	90%	81%	87%	85%
Some	10%	19%	13%	15%

	Rural (N=20)	Semi-rural (N=74)	Urban (N=86)	Total (N=180)
V-38 Prepares child for school by teaching:				
ABC or 1-2-3	31%	57%	84%	69%
Other	31%	29%	27%	28%
V-39 Mother structures observed play session	25%	27%	42%	34%
V-40 Mother's reaction when given toy for child				
Puts toy away without showing	5%	3%	4%	3%
Shows child without giving	5%	4%	6%	5%
Gives to child	90%	93%	91%	92%
Mother's reaction when given book for child:				
Shows child book with enthusiasm (points to:				
ABC or pictures by name	22%	19%	31%	25%
Verbalizes to child about book, without pointing to content	22%	49%	38%	41%
Positions or directs child to look at book, without speaking	28%	10%	14%	14%
Holds book without showing it	28%	7%	15%	13%
Puts book down	0%	13%	3%	7%
Book was held in position for child's viewing	78%	80%	86%	83%
Child was allowed to touch book	72%	62%	59%	62%

1. Figures are taken from Home Scale Item I-1, number of times mother spoke spontaneously to the child.

Construction of LAGOS HOME Scales

Using both the questions designed for the HOME Inventory and other interactional measures in the questionnaire, five scales that may serve as a starting point for further work on an instrument for assessing the home environment in Nigeria were constructed.

Criteria for selection of variables

The construction began with factor analysis to detect underlying dimensions. Then among the variables revealed by the factor analysis, a selection was made based on the following criteria:

(i)   theoretical relevance to child development outcomes,

(ii)   actual power to differentiate between high- and low-scoring and well- and malnourished children,

(iii)   performance of the variable in Kuder-Richardson reliability analyses, and

(iv)   ease with which a field worker could score the variable in a brief and unobtrusive home visit.

Table 12.15: Opportunities for variety
HOME SCALE VI by location

Means (SD) Percentages

	Rural (N=20)	Semi-rural (N=74)	Urban (N=86)	Total (N=180)
VI-41 Father and another male relative plays with child daily	95%	88%	94%	92%
V-42 Someone reads or recites with child	25%	20%	17%	19%
His *oriki*	755	91%	86%	87%
Stories	15%	35%	45%	37%
Songs or verses	80%	85%	91%	87%
VI-43 Childs eats with mother and father at least three times a week	45%	53%	61%	56%
VI-44 Child is taken to house of relatives or friends at least once a week	60%	46%	32%	41%
VI-45 Child owns more than two books of his own	33%	15%	10%	14%
Number of books owned by child	5(9.2)	2(6.1)	1(4.2)	2(5.8)
VI-46 Children in family have started going to lessons	58%	66%	92%	78%
Older sibling	10%	4%	12%	8%
Index child				

Almost all the variables were binary. Some dimensions were not represented and consequently these aspects could not be measured.

Dimensions not measured

At least three important dimensions were either not represented in a form suitable to use in a home inventory, or not represented at all. One of these is the verbal responsivity scale. While measures do exist for this dimension below, we lack good variables for the mother's spontaneous verbalizations to the child, and for her labelling of objects, probably because the HOME observation occurred with the Bayley testing although the ethnography provides evidence for the importance of both these items.

Table 12.16: Toys and tasks by location

Percentages

	Rural (N=20)	Semi-rural (N=74)	Urban (N=86)	Total (N=180)
Total number of manufactured toys				
0	60%	52%	38%	47%
1-2	25%	39%	50%	43%
3-4	15%	8%	12%	11%
Total number of non-manufactured toys				
0	20%	15%	17%	17%
1-2	55%	45%	57%	52%
≥3	25%	40%	26%	32%
Total number of children's books (picture books, story books, picture calendars)				
≤1	80%	54%	41%	51%
≥2	20%	46%	59%	49%
Total number of school books (textbooks and exercise books)				
0	45%	38%	26%	33%
≥1	55%	62%	74%	67%
Number of chores performed by child (housework, washing cup, buying things)				
≤1	70%	53%	51%	54%
2	20%	30%	30%	33%
3	2%	12%	18%	13%
Number of self-help tasks performed by the child (puts own things away, washes hands)				
0	5%	3%	1%	2%
1	15%	13%	8%	10%
2	80%	84%	93%	88%
Two or more things owned by child (cup and spoon, chair, crib, bed)	45%	43%	54%	49%

Another dimension was adequacy of alternative child care arrangements. The data set probably contains adequate information to create a child care and social variety inventory scale but such a scale would require careful thought, however, because the children whose mothers take them to work have the highest number of outings, although this was not positive for nutritional or developmental outcomes when the child remained tied to the back.

Yet another dimension which may be important but for which we had no adequate measure is the degree to which the environment offers the space and opportunity for the child to explore and process stimuli thoughtfully.

Table 12.17: Mother's emotional and verbal responsivity
Home Scale 1 by developmental group

Percentages

	Low (N=69)	High (N=69)
I-1 Number of times mother spontaneously spoke to child		
None	42%	43%
One	13%	10%
Two	20%	22%
Three or more	12%	12%
I-2 Mother's verbal response to child's verbalizations		
Made non-verbal sounds		
Sometimes	6%	10%
Usually	1%	7%
Used simple words the child could repeat		
Sometimes	29%	45%
Usually	6%	16%
I-3 Told child the name of an object		
Sometimes	59%	59%
Usually	39%	41%
I-4 Speech was audible and clear	99%	97%
I-5 Started a conversation with field workers	65%	71%
I-6 Conversed freely and easily with field workers	6%	13%
I-7 Let child play with "messy mud, water, Sand	56%	44%
I-8 Spontaneously praised child at least twice	64%	51%
I-9 Conveyed positive feelings toward child by tone of voice	14%	13%
I-10 Caressed or kissed child at least once	52%	43%
I-11 Responded positively to praise of child		

Draft Lagos HOME Scales

The draft scales shown below incorporate very few variables which are important but for which there is little variability because almost all the children do them or have them, e.g. recitation of the *oriki*, and playing on a pretend musical instrument. In further revision, it would be desirable to include these because they would assist in detecting the few children for whom the usual cultural supports do not operate.

Table 12.18: Mother's acceptance of child's behaviour
Home Scale II by developmental group

Means (SD) Percentages

	Low (N=69)	High (N=69)
II-12 Shouted at child	46%	54%
II-13 Expressed annoyance or hostility	9%	13%
II-14 Slapped or spanked child	9%	12%
II-15 Said child does not usually obey, requires punishment		
Said child needed spanking –	18%	25%
Never	18%	15%
More than once a week, but less than daily	71%	73%
Many times a week, can't remember exactly	11%	12%
II-16 Scolds or criticizes the child	17%	14%
II-17 Did not interfere with or restrict the child more than three times	97%	100%
II-18 Visual reading or teaching materials in home		
Number of books in home	3.5(2.3)	4.3(2.2)
Picture books	47%	54%
Story books	35%	52%
Picture calendars	78%	87%
Magazines with pictures	38%	41%
ABC or 1, 2, 3, book	50%	54%
Older child's school books	51%	77%
School notebooks	54%	68%
II-19 Pet cat or dog in home		
None	82%	74%
Present, child not allowed to play with	3%	4%
Present, child allowed to play with	15%	22%

Discussion of the scales

(1) Verbal responsivity
This scale measures whether the mother responded to the child's vocalizations with repeatable short words or nonsense sounds, or gave no response or a response using adult speech. It also represents her fluency and initiative in interacting with the field workers.

Table 12.19: Organization of the Environment
Home Scale III by developmental group

Percentages

	Low (N=69)	High (N=69)
III-20 Child has 1-3 Primary caretakers	88%	93%
III-21 Child accompanies mother every work to:		
Market	25%	20%
Shops	36%	37%
Church	59%	62%
Mosque	19%	15%
House of friends or relatives	47%	38%
III-22 Child usually accompanies mother to work	53%	47%
Total number of outings per week child accompanies mother		
0	13%	17%
1-2	56%	54%
3-4	27%	23%
5-6	4%	6%
III-23 Number of times child taken for check-up when not ill.		
0-7	64%	77%
≥8	36%	23%
III-24 Child has special spaces to keep toys or treasures	52%	48%
III-25 Child's play environment is safe	78%	66%

This scale was found to correlate significantly and positively with all of the child developmental measures and also with the Extended Parental Protection and Manufactured toy scales (see below), the mother's use of family planning, whether any of her children died, birth interval, and with the composite quality-of-child-care scale. It correlates significantly and negatively with the mother's per capita earnings and, after controlling for the child's age and birth interval, with the ratio of the mother's earnings to the father's contribution to food expenditure. It also was marginally negative (Spearman p=.077) with the family's score on the farming scale.

(2) Teaching play
This scale correlated positively with mental development but not with the nutritional variables. It suggests that children whose more highly educated parents were teaching them ABC's and reading to them, had

shorter birth intervals and were marginally lower in weight-for-age than those whose parents were not so educated.

Table 12-20: Provision of play materials
Home Scale IV by developmental group

Percentages

	Low (N=69)	High (N=69)
IV-31 Child has own-		
cup, plate, or spoon	82%	74%
chair	50%	62%
Crib or bed	3%	14%
IV-32 Manufactured toys		
Football	7%	145
Plastic ball	6%	9%
Wheeled toy to sit on	3%	6%
Rocking horse	4%	9%
Toy car	3%	6%
Toy plane	0%	3%
Wind-up toy	0%	0%
Plastic doll	16%	17%
Plastic rattle	4%	12%
Blocks	0%	0%
Plastic building toys "legos"	0%	0%
Real or toy musical instrument	18%	19%
Teddy bear, other stuffed animal	0%	3%
Other toys	11%	20%
IV-33 Homemade toys		
Bottle covers	22%	20%
Special stones, sticks	25%	23%
Empty tins	53%	49%
Plastic cups, other plastic containers	34%	23%
School box	3%	1%
Paper or newspaper	12%	10%
Plastic bag	13%	4%
Special cloth	1%	7%
Pretend musical instrument	91%	96%
Sand or mud	29%	29%
Water	13%	9%
Games	31%	20%

This is also the only scale that was significantly associated with the sex of the child, with girls scoring higher. The mothers of girls also had been rated significantly higher in the warmth/rewarding scale of the behaviour and affect ratings. The scale was highly positive with the

scales for books and pictures and manufactured toys, the food investment
scale, the belief that giving meat would not spoil the child's moral
training, the father's contribution to food expenditure, use of family
planning, parental schooling (Spearman r = .41 with a composite of
mother's schooling and current events knowledge), with the behaviour
and affect rating that she was warm/rewarding and with the urban end of
all of the urbanization measures. Conversely the scale was negative with
ties to agriculture, experience of child death in the family, and illness of
the index child, and only marginally positive with the Extended Parental
Protection scale.

Table 12.21: Parental involvement
Home Scale V by developmental group
Percentages

	Low (N=69)	High (N=69)
V-35 Mother keeps child in visual range, looks at often	70%	87%
Mother plays with child		
Engages in social play	98%	99%
Technical play with toys or objects	6%	15%
Socio-technical play, including social interaction and objects	25%	34%
V-36 Parent talks to child while doing housework		
Never	42%	43%
One	13%	10%
Twice	20%	22%
Three or more times	12%	12%
V-37 Has taught child to:		
Take things from one place to another	100%	100%
Carry water in a small bowl	94%	97%
Wash one plate or cup	43%	41%
Put own thins away	90%	99%
Buy things	94%	96%
Do housework (e.g. sweeping, washing clothes)	69%	77%
Number of different chores performed by child		
None	78%	85%
Some	72%	14%
V-38 Prepares child for school by teaching:		
ABC or 1-2-3	74%	72%
Other	42%	18%
V-39 Mother structures observed play session	36%	33%

	Low (N=69)	High (N=69)
V-40 Mother's reaction when given toy for child:		
Puts toy away without showing child	3%	1%
Shows child without giving	6%	3%
Gives to child	91%	96%
Mother's reaction when given book for child:		
Shows child book with enthusiasm (points to		
ABC or pictures by name	27%	27%
Verbalizes to child about book, without pointing to content	52%	42%
Positions or directs child to look at book, without speaking	12%	14%
Holds book without showing it	7%	9%
Puts book down	3%	8%
Book was held in position for child's viewing	80%	83%
Child was allowed to touch book	61%	60%

1. Figures are taken from Home Scale I-1, number of times mother spoke spontaneously to the child

(3) Manufactured toys

This scale combines the provision of manufactured toys with the possession of a crib or chair for the child. The maximum score of any child on this scale was 8, making it comparable in dimensions with the other scales. In fact a child may learn just as much from improvised toys as from manufactured toys. In our data set, however, mothers who mentioned and showed the interviewers improvised play materials, had children who were worse off developmentally than those who did not. It may have been a point of pride to mention and show only manufactured playthings. Certainly possession of purchased toys is a measure of investment in the child and of the value attached by the parents to the child's play.

This scale had the highest correlations with all of the developmental measures as well as with food investment. It was significant and positive with all of the other scales, with a variant form of the verbal scale measuring only mother's responsiveness to child's vocalizations, and with the father's contribution to food expenditure, monogamy, use of family planning (now and ever), good quality of child care, mother's education, urbanization, a warm rewarding mother and the attractiveness of the child. It was significant and negative with child's illness, duration of breast-feeding and total household members, as to be expected.

(4) Books and pictures

This scale combines children's books, magazines, etc., with school books and exercise books. It correlates only marginally with nutritional outcomes for the same reason as the teaching scale, since the ABC books and picture books had the same paradoxical relationship with WAZ as the teaching of the ABC's and reading to the child. By contrast, the presence of older children's books was significant and positive with nutrition but less so with the Bayley score.

Table 12.22: Opportunities for variety
Home Scale VI by developmental group

Percentages

	Low (N=69)	High (N=69)
VI-41 Father and another male relative plays with child daily	85%	94%
V-42 Someone reads or recites with child		
his oriki	91%	94%
Stories	43%	39%
Sons or verses	93%	87%
VI-43 Child eats with mother and father at least three times a week	43%	61%
VI-44 Child is taken to house of relatives or friends at least once a week	47%	38%
VI-45 Child owns two or more books of his own	9%	10%
VI-46 Children in family have started going to lessons		
Older sibling	78%	82%
Index child	9%	12%

The books and pictures scale was significant and positive with the MDI but not with the PDI. It correlated significantly with the mother's responsiveness to child vocalizations and Manufactured Toys scale. It did not correlate significantly with Extended Parental Protection and only marginally with food investment. It was positive with current family planning, parental education and urbanization, and also with the mother's age, her rating as warm/rewarding, her number of children, and the total of household members. It was negative with the farming scale.

(5) Extended parental protection
This scale tells a more complex story than the others. As visible in the Chronbach's alpha values in Table 12.27, the reliability of the scale is significantly higher for the well-nourished subgroup than for the systematic or total samples. We believe its very meaning is complicated by malnutrition.

Table 12.23: Toys and tasks by developmental group

Percentages

	Low (N=69)	High (N=69)
Total number of manufactured toys		
0	64%	41%
1-2	32%	43%
3-4	4%	16%
Total number of non-manufactured toys		
0	13%	22%
1-2	55%	49%
≥3	32%	29%
Total number of children's books (picture books, Story books, picture calendars)		
≤1	54%	38%
≥2	46%	62%
Total number of school books (textbooks And exercise books)		
0	46%	23%
≥1	54%	77%
Number of Chores performed by child (housework, Washing cup, buying things)		
≤1	57%	50%
2	23%	35%
3	19%	14%
Number of self-help tasks performed by the child (puts own things many, washes hands)		
0	3%	0%
1	12%	6%
2	19%	94%
Two or more things owned by child (cup and spoon, chair, crib, bed)	47%	55%

The components of this scale are:
- the child stays close to the mother when the mother is working at home or near home,
- the child eats regularly with mother and with both parents,
- the mother openly caresses the child,
- she does not discipline with shouts or slaps,
- she does not teach/force the two-year-old to begin housework chores,
- she keeps the child in a safe play environment, and
- she takes child for health treatment to a Western-style clinic, nurse or doctor.

**Table 12.24: HOME Inventory Reference and subscale results for
the families of children studied in Nigerian surveys**

Means (SD)

	Study sample mean age 23.9 months	Caldwell sample mean age 24 months
I. Emotional and verbal responsivity	9.99(1.48)	8.47(1.99)
II. Acceptance of child's behaviour	5.84(1.35)	5.24(1.64)
III. Organization of environment	2.90(1.30)	4.93(1.24)
IV. Provision of play materials	4.23(1.43)	6.36(2.03)
V. Parental involvement with child	3.71(1.28)	354(1.79)
VI. Opportunities for variety	2.32(0.89)	3.03(1.52)
Total Score	28.91(4.58)	31.69(7.54)

A converse statement of the scale also is revealing:

- the child usually is off in the care of siblings or others,
- the child eats with siblings rather than parents, the mother is
  not expressively affectionate, but shows hostility and spanks if
  the child is disobedient, the child is expected to do housework,
- no special safe play area is provided for child,
- the child is taken for treatment primarily to traditional healers,
  herb stalls, or a pharmacy.

**Table 12.25: Reliability coefficients of Caldwell HOME inventory
subscales used with Nigerian families**

Subscales	Number of items	Alpha Values
I. Emotional and Verbal Responsivity	11	.10
II. Acceptance of Child's behavior	8	.45
III. Organization of Environment	6	.33
V. Provision of Play Materials	9	.36
V. Parental involvement with child	6	.19
VI. Opportunities for variety	5	.11
Total Score	6	.39

This converse statement appears to characterize the expected
transition of the two-year-old child in traditional African culture (LeVine
et al.; Omwana) to the lowest rung on the seniority ladder.

Confusion arises over the meaning of the more protected treatment
indicated by positive values on the Extended Parental Protection scale.

This is the type of treatment traditionally given to younger babies (LeVine *et al.*, 1990) and to sick babies, where infancy is viewed as a time of risk and the mother as a "folk paediatrician." Protective care previously reserved for young infants who had to be close to their mothers for breast-feeding and who were perceived during the first year of life to be at high mortality risk, now is being extended by urbanizing educated parents to their older toddlers.

Both Spearman and partial correlations, controlling for the children's four-month age variation around two years and birth interval of the child, yield a significant association between this scale and the death of previous children, together with a slight negative correlation with mother's age. Thus we see relatively younger mothers who have lost previous children protecting a subsequent child more carefully.

The scale is positive and significant with the Verbal Responsivity and Manufactured Toy scales and with food investment, marginally positive with Teaching Play, but not significant with Books and Pictures. The scale is strongly positive with all measures of urbanization, with the presence of the father living with the family, and with Christian rather than Muslim religious affiliation. Yet, when controlling only for age and birth interval, we observe no significance between the Extended Parental Protection scale and any of the outcome indicators except for the MDI (partial r =.2, p=.018).

In an attempt to remove the effects of perceived negative risk factors that would persuade parents to protect this particular child more carefully, we ran a partial correlation controlling for age, illness history, WAZ, and number of previous children who had died. Positive associations emerged with arm circumference (r=.18, p=.029) and with WHZ (r=.17,p=.04) but not with HAZ or WAZ. This indicates that the children given Extended Parental Protection were better nourished for their height, but not taller, a finding consistent with their significantly shorter birth intervals (r=.23, p=.0005) and younger (r=-.18, p=.007).

The fathers of extended protection children had significantly more education (r=.15, p=.02) and provided significantly more food money (r=.13, p=.04); and the ratio of the mother's earnings to this amount was lower (r=-.12, p=.068). Their mothers were significantly higher on the media and education exposure scale (r=.13, p=.033) though only marginally higher on education as such. The children's duration of breast-feeding also was significantly shorter (r=-.17, p=.01) and the correlation with short birth interval increased (r=-.27, p=.002).

In the presence of these controls, the scale's correlations with MDI, the co-operative child rating, and the Teaching Play scale increased.

Table 12.26: Draft Simplified Lagos HOME scales

1.Verbal responsivity of parent
Responds to child's verbalization
with nonsense sounds   1.___
   never (0)   2.___
   sometimes (1)
   usually (2)
with simple words child can repeat 3.___
   never (0)   4.___
   sometimes (1)   5.___
   usually (2)   6.___
Starts conversion with tester
Converses freely, easily with tester

II. Teaching play   7.___
Parent teaches child   8.___
  ABC 123   9.___
  To wash own hands and face
  To put own things away   10.___
Parent sits and plays with child
with toys and objects (technical   11.___
play)
Combining social play and objects 12.___
socio-technical play)   13.___
Someone reads to the child from a
book   14.___
Someone tells child stories   15.___
                                   16.___
III. Manufactured toys   17.___
Child has manufactured   18.___
  Football   19.___
  Plastic ball   20.___
  Wheeled toy to sit on   21.___
  Rocking horse   22.___
  Toy car
  Toy plane
  Plastic rattle
  Plastic doll   23.___
  Plastic building toys   24.___
  Fit-together bricks   25.___
  Teddy bear, stuffed animal
  Special cloth
  Other purchased toys   26.___
Child has own furniture
  Chair   27.___
  Crib or bed

IV. Books and Pictures
Home has
  ABC or 123 Book   28.___
  Picture books   29.___
  Story books   30.___
  Picture calendars   31.___
  Magazines with pictures   32.___
Older child on have
  School textbooks   33.___
  School exercise books   34.___

V. Extended Parental
Protection
When mother working near or
in home, child usually stay with
her or in her sight   35.___
Child eats twice weekly or
more with
  mother   36.___
  mother and father   37.___
Parent says child minds well,
  does not express any
hostility,   38.___
  does not shout, slap or
  verbally threaten child   39.___
Parent has not taught child to   40.___
Do housework such as
  sweeping, washing clothes,
  wash own plate or cup   41.___
Play environment is safe   42.___
Parent takes child to modern
health care   43.___

Table 12.27: Reliability of draft Lagos HOME scales

		Samples	
	Total	Systematic	Well-nourished
1.Verbal Responsivity			
Items 1-6			
Chronbach's ALPHA	.23	.16	.06
Standardized item	.24	.13	.00
Without item 5			
Chronbach's ALPHA	.49	.40	.40
Standardized item	.40	.38	.38
II. Teaching play			
Chronbach's ALPHA	.53	.53	.47
Standardized item	.53	.54	.44
III. Manufactured Toys			
Items 14-27			
Chronbach's ALPHA	.22	.20	.19
Standardized item	.27	.25	.23
Without items 26-27			
Chronbach's ALPHA	.40	.38	.41
Standardized item	.41	.39	.43
IV. Books and pictures			
Items 28-34			
Chronbach's ALPHA	.71	.71	.69
Standardized item	.68	.68	.65
Without items 33-34, about .80			
V. Extended parental protection			
Items 35-43			
Chronbach's ALPHA	.34	.33	.47
Standardized item	.22	.35	.47
Without item 36, about 4.02			

Discussion of the extended parental protection scale

An alternative name for the Extended Parental Protection scale could be the Companionship scale. The dimension measured fits well with the progression of urbanization first described in Nigeria and Ghana by Caldwell (1977), as "a movement toward monogamy, a strengthening of the conjugal bond over all others, a strengthening of the parent-child bond over all relationships external to the nuclear family, and ultimately an emphasis on what parents owe children rather than what children owe parents."

Our choice of the word companionship to characterize the closer parent-child bond draws on the derivation of the word companion - one with whom one eats bread - and its connotations of friendship, warmth and security.

Of particular interest is the fact that Caldwell was writing primarily about the middle class. Although the Extended Parental Protection scale is significantly correlated with education and the income expenditure variables in our sample, these correlations are not high. Moreover, our sample was deliberately chosen from low-income neighbourhoods, and could therefore not be characterized as middle class by wealth criteria.

This suggests that a process of secular change is currently expanding values held primarily by the middle class in the 1970s to low-income urban dwellers as well. It may also confirm Caldwell's conclusion,

> if economic change were to be halted now, the crumbling [of the old social order] would continue.

Our findings regarding secular change are remarkably congruent with a primarily American-based literature of the 1960s (Becker, 1964; Bronfenbrenner, 1960, 1963) showing that middle class parents provide more warmth to their children, are more permissive, and use reasoning and appeal to the child's emotions of guilt, for example, to discipline them. These secular trends (summarized by LeVine, 1967) included greater acceptance of the child's spontaneous desires, and freer expression of affection. In contrast, the working class ridicule, shout, physically punish, or restrict the children.

This literature also indicates that U.S. secular trends across classes in the 1930s tended to shift in the direction of what had been predominantly middle-class values and techniques, leading to a narrowing of the gap between social classes in their patterns of child rearing.

These changes led in succeeding generations to shifts in the relative position of the father and the mother, with the former becoming increasingly more affectionate and less authoritarian and the latter becoming relatively more important as the agent of discipline, especially for boys.

Our findings also are remarkably similar to those of LeVine (1967), who compared a small ethnographic sample of elite Ibadan Yoruba families with more traditional families from Oje, a nearby market community. LeVine found fewer household tasks assigned by the father to a child among the elite, as well as greater paternal warmth ratings, contrasted with a tendency for more physical forms of punishment and less tolerance of the child's aggression on the part of the Oje market fathers.

In contrasting the same ethnographic samples (of about 30 in each group), Lloyd (1970) found that 90% of the elite versus 50% of the market mothers wanted immediate, as contrasted to qualified, obedience from their children. Only 3% of the elite vs. 55% of the market mothers mentioned errands as their first expectation of the well-behaved child. Market women's concerns were with "obedience and responsibility learning" while the elite placed an emphasis on intellectual achievement and self-reliance.

Our interpretation of the resemblance of these shifts across time and across culture is that similar social conditions of production in the global marketplace (as best this "marketplace" is approximated from country to country) evoke similar shifts in parenting behaviours despite different starting points in traditional economies.

Association between selected aspects of nutritional status, home stimulation and cognitive performance

Associations between the LAGOS HOME Scale and Food Restriction

Parents who scored high on the overall LAGOS HOME and on the subscales tended to score significantly higher on the food investment variable, and lower on a composite scale of negative beliefs that meat would spoil the child's moral character, cause him to steal, or spoil him for scarcity. However, the very nature of the protective concept may lead in practice to a prolonging of the food taboos of infancy with regard to animal foods.

Cognitive scores and nutrition

Overall, the Nigerian children in our sample generally tended to perform better on the perceptual-motor items than the reference American population on which the tests were standardized. These items, which were passed by 50% or more of the Nigerian children at an earlier age than the American standardization sample included:

- •tower building, train, pinkboard,
  which involves fitting the right geometric shapes into the appropriate holes even in the face of confusing cues and
- •   language comprehension,
  which involves discriminating between two or more objects. The child is presented with three different containers and the examiner asks him to bring one or the other to show that he understands.

Since the environment in which these children live is full of single-level dwellings, it is surprising that they should demonstrate a better understanding of 'tower-building'. It seems likely that the children may have learned by observing their parents, or perhaps have been specifically taught, a skill of putting things away in the limited space of their one-room homes by stacking them one on top of the other or as closely together as possible on limited floor space. Hence, too, they are able to make a 'train' of cubes in the Bayley test.

The mothers probably encourage receptive language, as tested by the language comprehension activity, because it is important for the children to understand the parents' commands. Many of the mothers sent the two-year-olds on errands around the house, and expected the children to be able to distinguish which object the mother wanted them to bring.

We found in this study that most of the children were not able to pass items in the Bayley Scales which had to do with naming objects, naming and recognizing pictures, and pointing to and identifying pictures in a book. Performance on these items was worse than for the reference sample. These items require that the children "speak out" or produce language when the examiners ask them to do so. Their failure on these items may be due in part to shyness. But many also were not familiar with the pictures of the objects they had to name, such as the American flag, or a clock.

However, among those children who were able to pass the productive language items which most of the sample failed, it was found that what made the difference was the home availability of various kinds of books (including picture books, calendars, magazines, story books, exercise books, etc.); mothers spending time with the children teaching ABC, 123; mothers playing with the children using manufactured toys, and the mother's emotional attitude towards the child as assessed by whether she encouraged him or her to perform on the Bayley test by empathizing, comforting, guiding, managing the child well, and showing visible pleasure in the child's achievements and obvious disappointment when she or he failed. Also found to be significant was the amount of time that the child's father spent in the home and his financial contribution.

While these factors in the child's home environment are important, it seems likely that more distal socio-economic factors are also relevant and possibly determine the absence or presence of some of these home stimulation variables. For example, the family income determines whether the family can afford manufactured toys for the child or more meat in the diet. Similarly, mothers who have greater exposure to media and who live in better quality housing with good electricity and water supply tend to show more eagerness and emotional support for the child in a testing situation. In other words, the mother's socio-economic status and living conditions affects her emotional state and the amount of enthusiasm and emotional encouragement which she can pass on to the child to stimulate performance.

Comparison of malnourished and well nourished children

It is not only general mental development that may be affected by malnutrition. The findings of the present study show that specific cognitive skills, especially those that involve perceptual-motor (eye-hand) co-ordination, puzzles, pre-writing skills, language comprehension and the understanding of prepositions were most significantly depressed in the presence of malnutrition.

T-test comparisons of a better nourished group (1 SD above the sample mean) with a malnourished group (1 SD below the sample mean) showed highly significant differences between the two groups in these specific skills:

blue board	$p < .006$
pegboard	$p < .001$
pinkboard	$p < .02$
writing	$p < .01$
language comprehension	$p < .05$
understanding prepositions	$p < .05$

These skills are crucial for basic school learning, and delay in their acquisition at this vulnerable age implies that the malnourished children may already be cognitively disadvantaged in preparation for school.

The findings of this project show that malnourished children are not usually started on domestic tasks at age two ($r = .25$, $p < .001$). Some of these activities have been found to be significantly associated with the child's overall mental development and specific cognitive skills. For example, the encouragement of self-help skills in the child, such as putting his own things away and washing his own hands, correlated significantly with higher general mental development ($r=.25$, $p<.001$) and with specific aspects of the Bayley Mental Development Scales such as the pink board ($p<.02$), the perceptual-motor scale ($p<.05$), and the language comprehension scale ($p<.028$).

Because the malnourished child is physically weak, parents seem not to encourage him to do things for himself or to help with small tasks around the house. Since these mothers are usually so busy, the only interactions they have with their children tend to be in the context of getting the children to help them with their household tasks, some of which appear to be beneficial for stimulating the development of skills which emphasize inter-sensory co-ordination, problem-solving, and productive language as well as responsibility training and personal effectiveness.

Whether well nourished or malnourished, children need specific kinds of stimulation and information in order to stimulate their mental development. The malnourished child may miss out on the limited opportunities which his environment provides for adult-child interaction. However, the adverse effects of malnutrition may be reduced if the children are growing up in an environment which is educationally stimulating. Conversely, no matter how well nourished children are, they will not develop particular mental skills if their environmental experiences do not provide them with the necessary context and inputs which would develop such skills.

Glossary

Agbo – herbal decoction
Ayanmo – destiny
Akara – fried beans cake
Amala – food made from yams
Apon – seeds of a fruit, crushed and cooked
Babalawo – traditional medicine man
Eba – food made from processed cassava
Efirin – spicy herb used in stews with medicinal quality to clear upset stomach
    and heart-burn
Egbo – maize porridge
Egungun – bogeyman - traditional masquerade
Egusi – melon seeds
Eko – solid maize pap
Eko jiji – cold pap
Eko mimu – hot pap
Elubo – yam powder usually prepared into a staple plate
Ewa – beans
Ewedu – a slippery leafy green vegetable
Fufu – ready to eat i.e. cooked cassava wrapped in leaves
Gari – meal processed from cassava
Gbegiri – bean soup
Ikokore – meal made of yam
Isoye – powdered herbal concoction said to improve memory
Kokoro – insect in food e.g. weevils in beans
Kuli-kuli – ground nut snack?
Lafun – food made from cassava
Manu – a snack food
Moinmoin – steamed beans cake
Nisin – recently, now, now-a-days
Obeewuro – bitter leaf soup
Ogi – fermented, diluted, white maize pap
Oriki – praise poem specific to family containing key characteristics of lineage
Orisha – the pantheon of Yoruba divinities
Osun – red mud used both as cosmetics and antiseptic for rash

Otili – small beans
Ponmo – cow hide, processed and cooked
Robo – groundnut cake from which the oil has been extracted
Seke – plantain soaked in red palm oil, a snack food
Sese – small fish
Suya – pieces of beef grilled, beef kebabs
Tuwo – a meal prepared from millet, maize or rice
Wara – seasoned and solidified sour milk, a kind of cheese
Wuwo – a term used to describe an immobile, heavy older infant

Bibliography

Adebayo, A, 'The masculine side of planned parenthood: an explanatory analysis,' *Journal of Comparative Family Studies* 18(1) 1988

Adenike, A., *et al.* 'Anthropometry and nutrient intake of Nigerian school children from different ecological zones', *Ecology of Food and Nutrition,* 21: 271-285, 1988

Adewale, S.A, 'Ethics in Ifa,' in Abogunrin, S.O. (ed.), *Religion and Ethics in Nigeria.* Ibadan, Nigeria: Daystar Press, 1986:60-71.

Agiobu-Kemmer, I, 'Cognitive and affective aspects of infant development,' Chapter 4 in Curran, H. V. (ed.) *Nigerian Children: Developmental Perspectives,* Boston: Rutledge and Kegan Paul, 1984.

Aina, T.A., Etta, F.E., and Zeitlin, M.F. (eds.) *Child Development and Nutrition in Nigeria: A Textbook for Education, Health and Social Service Professionals,* First Edition. Federal Government of Nigeria, Nigerian Education Research and Development Council and UNICEF Nigeria, 1992.

Aina, T.A., M. F. Zeitlin, L. Setiloane, and I. Agiobu-Kemmer, Positive Deviance in Nutrition Research Project, Lagos State, Nigeria: Phase I Survey Results, 1993.

Akinware, M., Wilson-Oyelaran, E.B., Ladipo, P.A., Pierce, D., and Zeitlin, M.F, 'Child Care and Development in Nigeria: A Profile of Five UNICEF Assisted LGA'S', Lagos: UNICEF Nigeria, 1992

Allen, L.H., Backstrand, J.R., Chavez, A., and Pelto, G.H., "People Cannot Live by Tortillas Alone: The Results of the Mexico Nutrition CRSP," Final Report to the U.S. Agency for International Development, Cooperative Agreement #DAN 1309-A-00-9090-00, University of Connecticut and Instituto Nacional de la Nutricion Salvador Zubiran, June 1992.

Annegers, J. A., 'Protein quality of West African foods' *Ecology of Food and Nutrition* 3: 125-130, 1974

Armstrong H., "Breastfeeding promotion; training of mid-level and outreach health workers." *International Journal of Gynecology and Obstetrics,* 1990; 31:91-103.

Armstrong, H.C., "International recommendations for consistent breastfeeding definitions." *J Hum Lact* 1991 7(2); 51-54

Atinmo, T. "Food problems and nutrition situation in Nigeria," in Atinmo, T. and Akinyele, O., eds., *Nutrition and Food Policy in Nigeria*. National Institute for Policy and Strategic Studies, Jos, 1983.

Babatunde, E. 'African culture: a definition', *Nigerian Journal of Theology, 4 (1), 1986.*

Babatunde, E.D. *Culture, Religion and the Self: A Critical Study of Bini and Yoruba Value Systems in Change*. New York: Mellen, 1992

Bascom, W.A, 'Yoruba food', *Africa*, 21: 40-53, 1951

Bayley, N. *Manual for the Bayley Scales of Infant Development*. New York: The Psychological Corporation, 1969.

Becker, W.C., Krug, R.S. A Circumplex Model for Social Behavior in Children. Child Development 1964; 35:391-396.

Boulding. E. *Building a Global Civic Culture: Education for an Interdependent World* Syracuse, New York: Syracuse University Press, 1990.

Bronfenbrenner, U. "The Changing American Child: A Speculative Analysis. In: Smelser, N.J., Smelser, W.T., eds. *Personality and Social System*. New York: Wiley, 1963.

Brown, L.V., Zeitlin, M.F., Peterson, K.E., Chowdhury, A.M.R., Rogers, B.L., Weld, L.H. and Gershoff, S.N., Evaluation of the Impact of Weaning Food Messages on Infant Feeding Practices and Child Growth in Rural Bangladesh. *American Journal of Clinical Nutrition.;*56:994-1003, 1992.

Caldwell, B.M., Bradley, R.H. *Home observation for measurement of the environment*, University of Arkansas, Little Rock, Arkansas, 1984.

Caldwell, J. C., Caldwell, P. 'High Fertility in Sub-Saharan Africa'*, Scientific American* May, 1990;118-125.

Caldwell, J.C. and Caldwell, P. The Economic Rationale of High Fertility: An Investigation Illustrated with Nigerian Survey Data. *Population Studies* 31:5-27, 1977.

Cassidy, C.M., World-View Conflict and Toddler Malnutrition: Change Agent Dilemmas, in Scheper-Hughes, N. (ed.) *Child Survival, Anthropological Perspectives on the Treatment and Maltreatment of Children*, Boston: Reidel, 1987. 293-324.

Castle, 'Maternal Attitude and Life Experience as Determinants of Child Care and Illness Management in Rural Mali'. Harvard Center for Population and Development Studies, Xerox draft, June 1992.

Cherian, A., Duggan, M.B., and Sterken, E, 'The epidemiology of malnutrition in young children in Zaria, Nigeria', *Ecology of Food and Nutrition,* 16: 1-12, 1985.

Chiang Mai Lactation Project, 'Breastfeeding practices in the developing world', International, *Journal of Gynecology and Obstetrics*, Supplement. 1: 129-132, 1989.

Cravioto, J., and Pericardia, E.R., 'Micro environmental Factors in Severe Protein Calorie Malnutrition' *Basic Life Sciences,* 7:25-35. 1976.

Danzinger, K, 'Parental Demands and Social Class in Java', *Indonesia. Journal of Social Psychology* 1960; 51:75-86.

Den Hartog, A.P, 'Unequal distribution of food within the household: a neglected aspect of food behavior', *FAO Nutrition Newsletter* 10(4): 8-17, 1972

Desai, S. 'Children at Risk: the Role of Family Structure in Latin America and West Africa', Paper prepared for presentation at the IFPRI - World Bank Conference on Intra-household Resource Allocation: Policies and Research Methods, 12-14 February 1992. IFPRI, Washington DC.

Dizard, J.E., Gadlin, H. *The Minimal Family*. Amherst, MA: University of Amherst Press, 1990.

Draper, H. H ; 'Biological, cultural and social determinants of nutritional status', in: Liederman, P. H. ; Tulkin, S. R and Rosenfield, A. eds. *Culture and infancy: Variations in the Human Experience, New York,* Academic Press, 1977.

Ebomoyi, E, 'A Comparative study of the nutritional status of children in urban and rural areas in Kwara state, Nigeria,' *Ecology of Food and Nutrition,* 19: 19-30; 1986.

Ekeh, P. *Colonialism and Social Structure*. Inaugural Lecture, Ibadan, University of Ibadan Press, 1982.

Enwemeka, O.S., Adeghe, N. U.; 'Some family problems associated with the presence of a child with handicap in Nigeria', *Child Care, Health and Development* 8(3) 1982.

Enwonwu, C.O, 'A review of nutrient requirements and nutritional status in Nigeria' In Atinmo, T. and Akinyele, O., eds., *Nutrition and Food Policy in Nigeria.* Jos: National Institute for Policy and Strategic Studies, 1983

Fadipe, N.A. *The Sociology of the Yoruba.* Ibadan: Ibadan University Press, 1970.

FAO, 'Caring for the socio-economically deprived and nutritionally vulnerable, Major issues for nutrition strategies', Theme paper No. 3, Rome: International Conference on Nutrition, 1992.

FAO/WHO/UNU Expert Consultation. *Energy and protein requirements,* World health Organization Technical Report Series 724; Geneva, 1985.

Federal Republic of Nigeria and UNICEF. *Children and Women in Nigeria: a situation analysis*. Lagos: Federal Government and UNICEF, 1990.

Golden, M.V., 'Sustainable Agriculture: Definition and Terms', Special Reference Briefs: SRB 94-05. National Agricultural Library, Beltsville MD 20705-2351, May 1994; 2-39.

Grindal, B, *Growing Up in Two Worlds: Education and Transition Among the Sisala of Northern Ghana*. New York: Holt, Rinehart and Winston, 1972.

Guldan. G.S., Zeitlin, M.F., Super, C.M., and Beiser, A., 'Maternal Education and Child Feeding Practices in Rural Bangladesh', *Social Science and Medicine*; 36(7):925-935, 1993.

Gurney, J., and Omololu, A.; 'A nutritional survey in South-Western Nigeria: the anthropometric and clinical findings,' *Environmental Child Health* 17(2): 50-61, 1971

Guyer, J.I. 'Changing Nuptiality in a Nigerian Community: Observations from the Field,' *Working Papers in African Studies*, No. 146. African Studies Center, Boston University, 270 Bay State Road, Boston, MA 02215, 1990.

Harkness S. and C. Super, 'The Developmental Niche: A Conceptualization at the Interface of Child and Culture,*"* *International Journal of Behavioral Development.* (9) 1987.

Hendrickse, R.G; 'Interactions of nutrition and infection: experience in Nigeria', in Wolstenholme, G, and O'Conner, M eds. *Nutrition and Infection,* CIBA Foundation Study Group, No.31, Little Brown, Boston, 1967.

Hoffman, L.W, 'Cross-Cultural Differences in Childrearing Goals', Chapter 9 in Levine, R.A., Miller, P.M. and West, M.M.(eds.) Parental Behavior in Diverse Societies, *New Directions for Child Development,* no. 40, San Francisco: Jossy-Bass, 1988. 99-122.

Ibukun-Olu, A., 'Classification of Nigerian foods: A review '; *Food and Nutrition Bulletin* 7: 59-63, 1984

Idusogie, E.O. and Olayide, S.O. 'Role of roots and tubers in Nigerian nutrition and agricultural development '; In Olayide, S.O, 'Role of roots and tubers in Nigerian nutrition and agricultural development,' in Olayide, S.O.(ed), *Food and Nutrition in Nigeria,* Ibadan University Press,1982.

Izuora, O.I., Ebigbo, P, 'Emotional reactions of adult Africans to children with severe kwashiorkor', *Child Abuse and Neglect* 7(3) 1983.

Jonsson, U. A Conceptual Analysis of Growth Monitoring and Promotion, Paper presented at the UNICEF Workshop on GMP Nairobi, 7-9 May 1992 and the IDRC Colloquium on Growth Promotion for Child Development Nyeri, 12-13 May 1992.

Kolasa, K.M, *The nutritional situation in Sierra Leone,* Report No. 1, Project on Consumption effects on economic policy; USAID contract: AID/DSAN-C-008.

Lepowsky, M.A., Food taboos, malaria and dietary change: infant feeding and cultural adaptation on a Papua New Guinea island,' *Ecology of Food and Nutrition 16:* 105-126, 1985.

LeVine R.A., Klein N.H., and Fries C.H. 'Father-child Relationships and Changing Life Styles in Ibadan', In: Miner, H., ed., *The City in Modern Africa.* New York: Praeger, 1967.

LeVine, R.A., Dixon, S., LeVine, S., Richman A., Leiderman, P.H., and Brazelton, T.B. *Omwana: Infants and Parents in a Kenya Community.* New York: Cambridge University Press, 1990.

Levine, R.A; 'Human Parental Care: Universal Goals, Cultural Strategies, Individual Behavior', Chapter 1 in Levine, R.A., Miller, P.M. and West, M.M.(eds.) *Parental Behavior in Diverse Societies*, New Directions for Child Development, no. 40, San Francisco: Jossey-Bass, 1988. 3-12.

LeVine, R.A; 'Parental goals: a cross-cultural view', *Teachers College Record* 76(2): 226-239, 1974.

Levi-Straus, C. *Structural Anthropology* University of Chicago Press, 1976.

Lloyd, B.B; 'Yoruba Mothers' Reports of Child-rearing, Some Theoretical and Methodological Considerations', in P. Mayer, ed. *Socialization; The Approach from Social Anthropology;* London, Tavistock, 1970.

Lloyd, B; 'Education in Family Life in the Development of Class Identification among the Yoruba', In: Lloyd, P.C., ed., *New Elites of Tropical Africa.* London: Oxford University Press, 1966.

Longhurst, R. Strategy for Care and Nutrition, Draft for Discussion, Nutrition Section, UNICEF, N.Y., July, 1993.

Matthews MK: Developing an instrument to assess infant breastfeeding behavior in the early neonatal period. Midwifery

Mead, M., *Culture and Commitment.* Garden City, New Jersey: Natural History Press, 1970.

Megawangi, R., Zeitlin, M.F., and Colletta, N.D., The Javanese Families, Chapter 6 in Zeitlin, M.F., and Megawangi, R., Kramer, E.M., Colletta, N.D. Babatunde, E.D., and Garman, D. *Strengthening the Family to Participate in Development,* Publication of the Social Sector Policy Analysis Project, operated by the Academy for Educational Development, U.S. AID, Bureau for Research and Development, Office of Education, January, 1993.

Mull, D.S. and J.D. 'Infanticide among the Tarahumara of the Mexican Sierra Madre,' in Sheper-Hughes, N. *Child Survival.* Dordrecht: Reidel, 1987

Nigeria Fertility Survey 1981/82 principal report. *World Fertility Survey International Statistical Institute.* Lagos: National Population Bureau, 1984

Odebiyi, A.I, 'Child rearing practices among nursing mothers in Ile Ife, Nigeria' ; *Child Care, Health and Development* 11(5) 1985

Ogbeide, O.; 'Nutritional hazards of food taboos and preferences in Mid-West Nigeria', *The American Journal of Clinical Nutrition :27 :213-216,1974.*

Ojofeitimi, E. O.; 'Partnership with fathers in combating malnutrition,' *Child Care, Health and Development* 10(2) 1984

Okeke, E.C. and Nweke, F.I. and Nnanyelugo, D.O ; ' The Consequences of Absence of Adult Males on the Nutritional Status of Members of Rural Farm Households: and Implications for Rural Development Programmes: A Case Study', , in Adekanye, T.O., *Women in Agriculture, Journal of the Institute of African Studies, University of Ibadan,* 1988. 69-71.

Olayide, S.O., and Olayemi, J. K.; 'Economic aspects of agriculture and nutrition: a Nigerian case study,' *Food and Nutrition Bulletin 1:* 32-38, 1978.

Onuoha, G.; 'The changing scene of food habits and beliefs among the Mbaise people of Nigeria; *Ecology of Food and Nutrition* 11: 245-250, 1982

Oyewole, A. I.; 'Home and School: effects of micro-ecology on children's educational achievement,' in Curran, H. (ed.) *Nigerian Children: Developmental Perspectives,* 1984.

Pelletier, D. L., 'The Uses and Limitations of Information in the Iringa Nutrition Program, Tanzania', *Working Paper* 5. Cornell Food and Nutrition Policy Program, 1991.

Ransome-Kuti O., *et al.,* 'Some socio-economic conditions predisposing to malnutrition in Lagos,' *Nigerian Medical Journal,* 2: 111-118, 1972.

Rea, J. N.; 'Social and economic influences on the growth of preschool children in Lagos,' *Human Biology* 43: 46-63, 1977

Scheper-Hughes, N., 'The Cultural Politics of Child Survival, Introduction', in Scheper-Hughes, N. (ed.) *Child Survival, Anthropological Perspectives on the Treatment and Maltreatment of Children*, Boston: Reidel, 1987, 1-29.

Scheper-Hughes, N., *Child Survival*, Dordrecht: Reidel, 1987

Scheper-Hughes, N; 'Social Indifference to Child Death,' *The Lancet*. Vol. 337: May 11, 1991, 1144-1147.

Scrimshaw, N.S., Taylor, C.E., Gordon, J. E., *Interactions of nutrition and infection*. WHO monograph series, no. 57, 1968

Setiloane, K., Intra-household Meat Distribution, Nutritional Need and Modernization among the Yoruba, Tufts University School of Nutrition, Ph.D. Thesis.

Simons, F. J., Traditional use and avoidance of foods of animal origin: a culture historical view. *Bioscience* 28: 178-184, 1978

Thomas, M. and Surachmad, W., 'Social Class Differences in Mothers' Expectations for Children in Indonesia.' *Journal of Social Psychology* 1952; 57:303-307.

Thompson, Barbara, 'The first fourteen days of some West African babies.' *The Lancet* ii: 40-45, 1966

Turnbull, C.M. Introduction: 'The African condition,' In Anthony, E.J., and Koupernik, C; *The Child in His Family; children at psychiatric risk*. Vol. 3, 227-245. New York: John Wiley and Sons, 1974.

Uchendu V.C. *The Igbo of Southeast Nigeria* New York: Holt, Rinehart and Winston, 1965, p. 62: For an unusual reason as well as because of the general scarcity of animal meat, children get little protein. The Igbo elders believe that a generous allowance of meat to a child may make him steal and be wasteful in later life.

Van Esterik, P. *Intra-family food distribution: its relevance for maternal and child nutrition ;* Paper prepared for the Maternal and Child Health Amendment to the Cornell Nutrition Surveillance Program, Ithaca, N.Y., March 1984

Vemury, M, 'Rural food habits in 6 developing countries: a study on environmental, social and cultural influence on food consumption patterns', *CARE,* New York, 1981.

Vemury, M., and Levine, H.; 'Beliefs and practices that affect food habits in developing countries: A literature review', *CARE,* New York, 1987.

Werner, E.E and R. Smith. *Vulnerable but Invincible, A Longitudinal Study of Resilient Children and Youth.* New York: McGraw Hill, 1982.

Werner, E.E. *Cross Cultural Child Development: A View from the Planet Earth.* Monterey, CA: Brooks Cole, 1979.

Whiten, A., Milner, P., 'The Educational Experiences of Nigerian Infants.' In: Curran, H.V., ed. *Nigerian Children: Developmental Perspectives*. Boston: Rutledge and Kegan Paul, 1984:34-73.

Whiting, B.B. and Whiting, J.W.M. *Children of Six Cultures, A Psycho-Cultural Analysis*. Cambridge, MA: Harvard University Press, 1975.

Wilson-Oyelaran, E.B. and Ladipo, P. *Child Care and Development, a Baseline Survey of Preschool Age Children in Owo Local Government*. UNICEF, Nigeria. July, 1988.

World Health Organization Technical Report Series 724; Geneva, 1985.

Zeitlin M.F. and Brown L.V., "Integrating Diet Quality and Food Safety into Household Food Security," Nutrition Consultants' Report Series ESN/CRS 91, Rome: FAO 1992.

Zeitlin M.F., Megawangi R., Kramer E.M., Colletta N.D., Babatunde E.D., and Garman D. *Strengthening the Family: Implications for International Development*. Tokyo: United Nations University Press. 1995.

Zeitlin, M., Super, C., Beiser, A., Guldan, G., Ahmed, N.U., Zeitlin, J., Ahmed, M. and Sockalingam, S., *A Behavioral Study of Positive Deviance in Young Child Nutrition and Health in Rural Bangladesh, Report to the Asia and Near East Bureau*, U.S. Agency for International Development, and the U.S. Office of International Health, October, 1989.

Zeitlin, M.F,. "Nutritional Resilience in a Hostile Environment: Positive Deviance in Child Nutrition." *Nutrition Reviews* 49(9), 259-268, 1991.

Zeitlin, M.F., Bonilla, J., Lamontagne, J. and Kramer, E.M., "Risk Factors Nutritional Stunting in Managua, Nicaragua," in draft for submission to *Social Science and Medicine*, 1992.

Zeitlin, M.F., G. Guldan, R.E. Klein, and N. Ahmed, "Sanitary Conditions of Crawling Infants in Rural Bangladesh" (Full-length version 75 pages; summary version 15 pages), Report to the AID Asia Bureau, Nov. 1985.

Zeitlin, M.F., Grange, A.O., Armstrong, H., and Annunziata, A.; 'The Age Scale.' *Journal of Tropical Pediatrics*:38, 52-54, 1992.

Zeitlin, M.F., H. Ghassemi, and M. Mansour, *Positive Deviance in Child Nutrition: with Emphasis on Psychosocial and Behavioral Aspects and Implications for Development*, Tokyo: The United Nations University, 1990.